Keto diet Cookbook Recipes

1000 Recipes
For Quick & Easy Low-Carb

The Complete Ketogenic Diet for Beginners

ASHLIE JACKSON

blame be held against the publisher for any reparation, damages, or monetary loss due to the information herein, either directly or indirectly.

Respective authors own all copyrights not held by the publisher.

The information herein is offered for informational purposes solely, and is universal as so. The presentation of the information is without contract or any type of guarantee assurance.

The trademarks that are used are without any consent, and the publication of the trademark is without permission or backing by the trademark owner. All trademarks and brands within this book are for clarifying purposes only and are the owned by the owners themselves, not affiliated with this document.

Disclaimer and Terms of Use: The Author and Publisher has strived to be as accurate and complete as possible in the creation of this book, notwithstanding the fact that he does not warrant or represent at any time that the contents within are accurate due to the rapidly changing nature of the Internet. While all attempts have been made to verify information provided in this publication, the Author and Publisher assumes no responsibility for errors, omissions, or contrary interpretation of the subject matter herein. Any perceived slights of specific persons, peoples, or organizations are unintentional. In practical advice books, like anything else in life, there are no guarantees of results. Readers are cautioned to rely on their own judgment about their individual circumstances and act accordingly. This book is not intended for use as a source of legal, medical, business, accounting or financial advice. All readers are advised to seek services of competent professionals in the legal, medical, business, accounting, and finance fields.

In this Piece I will be sharing with you some series of simple food-related Inventions, brilliant recipes of all kinds, the balance of contrasts in the kitchen.

SOMMARIO

Introduction

Save money and the food waste by using every part of the fruits and veggies you buy-including plenty of pieces that you usually throw away! These brilliant e-book recipes show you how and I bet you will be as amazed at some of those deliciously creative ideas!

Perhaps the most common cooking form, the barbecue is used in the world in the regional variations. It blossoms in the form of a tandoor in India, Turkey, Iran, Afghanistan, Pakistan, the Balkans, Central Asia, Burma and Bangladesh.

The tandoor is the accepted method of grilling in these parts of the world. The word "tandoor" is used to describe both the cylindrical clay oven used to cook and roast, and the cooking process itself.

The tandoor is said to have migrated along with the Roma or Romani people to Central Asia and the Middle East, also known as Gypsies to the Western world. Archeological evidence suggests the presence of the tandoor in the ancient Harappa and Mohenjo daro sites dating back as far as 3000 B.C. The tandoor's success in India continued through the times of Muslim rule in South Asia until the day the chicken tikka masala reigns supreme in restaurants around the world.

Traditionally, heat for the tandoor is produced by a charcoal or wood fire that burns inside the tandoor itself. Temperatures within the tandoor can approach up to 480°C (900°F) and it is not unusual for them to remain lit for long periods to maintain the high temperature.

Some types of Iranian, Afghan, Pakistani, and Indian dishes such as tandoori chicken, chicken tikka, and breads such as tandoori roti and naan, are the traditional foods cooked in the tandoor. The chicken tikka is a dish made in South Asia by grilling small pieces of chicken marinated with spices and yoghurt. It is traditionally boneless and cooked on the tandoor in skewers. It could be eaten like a kebab with green coriander chutney or could be used to prepare the curry chicken tikka masala.

The other favorite, tandoori chicken is a roasted delicacy that originated in North Western India. It later became a popular Punjabi dish during the time of the Mughals in Central and Southern Asia and remains popular in that area till date. The chicken is marinated in yoghurt seasoned with typically Indian spices such as garam masala, ginger, garlic, cumin, peppers, and turmeric for the red color. Cooked traditionally in the clay oven, it can also be done on a grill.

Like the barbecue itself, the tandoor's journey continues unceasingly, with Pakistani and Indian restaurants offering tandoori delicacies to countless visitors around the world. The tandoori repertoire has gone on to include all kinds of meats, seafood, poultry, vegetables, and even fruits and cheeses and its popularity continues to increase manifold everyday.

RECIPES 1: BITE SIZE CHICKEN TACOS-RECIPES FOR USING LEFTOVER CHICKEN

Are you still having a struggle trying to decide what to do with your chicken left over? Here are a couple of recipes to help you use the chicken left over!

It feels like there are still leftover rotisserie chicken in our room. One of my favorite stuff about making Chicken Tacos or Burritos is about this.

Chicken Style Tacos

1. Choose the leftover chicken from bone

2. Steam it up in a frying pan with taco seasoning and a limited amount of water (the guidelines on the taco seasoning packet can be followed).

3. Then make taco, or burrito, your favorite type.

I use soft shells, add a little lettuce, shredded cheddar cheese and some tomatoes. The flavor in these tacos is unbelievable! You can also make chicken fajitas this same way. Mmm...Mmmm...delicious!

One of the other things I love to do with leftover chicken is to make bbq chicken sandwiches.

BBQ Chicken Sandwich Recipe

1. Break the chicken into pcs and put in a small pan

2. Add enough of your favorite bbq sauce to coat the meat

3. Heat and serve on sandwich rolls.

That is what I call a quick and easy chicken dinner! The kids love these sandwiches served with french fries or mac and cheese.

Here are some of the best recipes for leftover chicken:

Easy Chicken Salad

You can use leftover rotisserie chicken or cooked chicken breast. They both taste great.

Ingredient quantities are left blank because the amounts will depend on how much chicken you are using. You can determine the amounts of each ingredient based on your taste.

Ingredients:

- o Cooked Chicken
- o Enough Mayo to coat chicken
- o Pinch of Salt
- o The following are all Optional Ingredients:
- o Sliced Celery
- o Chopped Onion
- o Small amount of chopped apple (cored and seeds removed)
- o Water chestnuts Pepper (to taste)

Tear or cut cooked chicken into bite size pcs. Combine Chicken with all ingredients except mayo. Add mayo after all other ingredients are combined. Chill before serving.

Sweet and Sour Chicken Stir-Fry

Ingredients:

- o 2 or 3 cooked boneless skinless chicken breast
- o 1 green bell pepper (slice into thin slices)
- o 1 clove of garlic (chopped or crushed)
- o 2 1/2 tbsp. of olive oil
- o 1 jar of La Choy sweet and sour sauce

Cube chicken into desired chunks; set aside.

Heat oil on low heat. Add garlic and bell pepper. Cook on low for about 5 minutes. Add sweet and sour sauce and chicken.

Cover and simmer for another 5 to 10 minutes until bell pepper is soft and tender and chicken is heated through. Serves 2-3.

Taco Salad Recipe for You

Those who have tried taco salad will agree that this salad is nutritious and delicious. It's colorful and crunchy with a zing. The new and vibrant flavors make it look so tempting that you'll try out more from men. One could often make this salad, and still want it to his or her family. And visitors are going to want to learn how to cook the salad. They'll all ask you to give them the special recipe for taco salads.

It is a very good recipe really. Any Chef will be pleased to share this with you. You should make the vegetarian or non-vegetarian salad according to your choice. The taco salad recipe that I will share with you is very simple and tasty. You can make it within minutes and add your own improvisations if you wish.

This is an excellent recipe by itself and does not require any correction. The meat that you are adding will rely on your taste. You can add raw boneless chicken, ground chuck or even rotting vegetarian beef. You'll need to procure the following ingredients to produce this excellent salad.

Ground Chuck/Boneless Chicken

- o Vegetarian meat crumbles - 1 lb
- o Milk - 1 cup
- o Garlic Powder - 1 tbsp
- o Chili Powder - 1 tbsp
- o Cumin - 2 tbsp
- o Salt & Pepper - to taste
- o Tortilla Chips (crushed) - 1 packet
- o Minced Garlic - 1 tbsp
- o Taco Cheese (shredded) - 1 packet
- o Hidden Valley Ranch dressing mix - 1 packet
- o Mayonnaise - 1 cup
- o Tomatoes (diced) - 3 large
- o Red/sweet onion (diced) - 1 Medium
- o Lettuce (chopped) - 1

Once you have the ingredients, follow the steps below for a wonderful taco salad.

1) Cook the meat for 5-10 minutes, first. Take some oil in a saucepan and prepare the seasonings with the meat. Connect the garlic, cumin, curry, salt and pepper

powder. Cook until the meat cooks well for about 10 minutes.

2) Mix all the vegetables in a big tub. With the ground garlic, mix them properly.

3) Combine the mayonnaise, milk and Secret Valley Ranch dressing together in another medium-sized pot. Place it back.

4) Smash the pieces of tortilla into the bag itself. Using a rolling pin and open a little end of the bag; gently smash the chips in the same bag.

5) Add the melted cheese and chips to a big veggy tub. Mix as well. Then apply the sauce and the meat and combine again.

Even children can make this salad under supervision of elders, of course. This salad, when ready, looks colorful with the greens of lettuce, reds of tomatoes, white from mayonnaise and cheese. It is juicy because of the added meat. The crunch of the chips makes every bite deliciously crunchy. There you have your bowl of some fantastic taco salad recipe, ready to be over within minutes! Make it once and take my word; your family and guests will love it. They will keep asking for more and you will have repeat requests to make this crunchy salad.

RECIPES 2: BUFFALO CHICKEN MOZZARELLA STICKS-BUFFALO CHICKEN PIZZA RECIPE

My family is a huge fan of buffalo and pizza wings but wings and kids can be messy! So to please both, I have come up with this simple but delicious recipe. Try this recipe and it will soon become a favorite of the household.

This Buffalo Chicken Pizza Recipe Uses:

- o Chicken marinated in a buffalo sauce
- o Blue cheese dressing instead of a red sauce
- o Two different types of cheeses
- o Your favorite toppings

Here's how we make ours, but to match your preferences, you can add or remove all of the toppings. If you like, instead of using the usual refrigerated crust, you can do your own recipe for pizza crust.

Ingredients:

- o 1 can (13.8 oz.) refrigerated pizza crust
- o 1 can (12.5 oz.) canned chicken, drained
- o 1/2 cup buffalo sauce

- o 2 Tablespoons of butter, melted
- o 1/2 cup Blue Cheese dressing
- o 1 cup Cheddar cheese
- o 1 cup Mozzarella cheese
- o 1 small red onion sliced
- o 1 cup real bacon bits
- o 1 cup banana peppers
- o Garlic powder
- o Onion powder
- o Salt

Directions:

Preheat oven to 220 ° C (450 ° F) Spray the non-stick cooking spray on an 11x15 inch pan. The chicken, hot sauce, and melted butter are mixed in a medium dish. Setting aside and letting marinate. Pat pizza dough in heated saucepan. Perforate the dough with a fork. Bake for another 5 minutes. Remove from the oven, and sprinkle dressing of blue cheese over pre-baked crust. Sprinkle over cheese. Place the chicken marinated over cheeses. Finish with red onion, authentic bacon bits and peppered bananas. Sprinkle on some ground garlic, onion powder, and butter. Start baking for another 8-12 minutes, or until golden brown is finished.

Make Buffalo Chicken Pizza

If a hot meal tickles your taste buds (and I'm not thinking about the temperature), then the chicken buffalo pizza is the best recipe you can know from. The buffalo chicken pie blends all the pie goodness into a sweet delicacy. It's a very simple recipe to follow and you will never go wrong with it. Preparing this pizza takes a relatively short time, and in no time do you and your family enjoy this savory and spicy treat.

The ingredients include melted butter, skinless and boneless chicken that has already been cubed, a container of blue cheese that is sometimes used as a salad sauce, a 16 inch chilled pizza crust, and a mozzarella cheese box. Cayenne pepper sauce can be used by those who want even more spice. All those ingredients can be found very easily. To cook this sort of pizza, you would require, of course, an oven and a baking pan, and a skillet. You will prepare everything you need in advance to ensure the cooking process runs smoothly

The steps for preparing the Buffalo Chicken Pizza are very simple and straightforward. First, pre-heat the oven at about 425 degrees Fahrenheit, or about 220 degrees Celsius. Then, you should unroll the pizza dough and put it in a lightly greased baking pan. The best baking pan should measure around fifteen inches, by ten inches, by one inch. Bake the dough for about seven minutes, and then remove it. You can then brush the dough with about two tablespoons of buffalo sauce. You should sprinkle the mozzarella cheese on top of the dough and then set it aside.

Take the cubed chicken and cook it separately in the skillet until the chicken pieces are no longer pink. You can spice it up with garlic, Cayenne pepper and salt. You should stir the chicken over medium heat in order to ensure that all the pieces are properly cooked. After the chicken has been properly prepared, you should spoon it over the pizza crust and cheese that you had prepared earlier.

Bake the pie for about eighteen to twenty minutes or until all the cheese has melted and the crust is light brown. You can opt to spice it up with blue cheese. This pie can be sliced into about eight slices, and can accommodate four people comfortably. You can be sure everybody will love this pizza and you can get a lot of orders for it to be made over and over. For some nutritious data, you will know that there are about three grams of fibre, 76 grams of protein and about 218 milligrams of cholesterol in one serving (which in our case is equivalent to two slices of pizza).

RECIPES 3: CREAMY SPINACH AND MUSHROOM-CREAMY RIGATONI FLORENTINE WITH SAUTEED MUSHROOMS AND TOASTED WALNUTS

Creamy Rigatoni Florentine is a rich and satisfying pasta dish with satiated mushrooms and toasted walnuts that combines the dry, earthy flavors of fall. Served as a vegetarian dinner, or as a side dish, this recipe is tasty, savory and nutritious. The recipe calls for button mushrooms-which are readily available in most grocery stores-and mascarpone cheese-an Italian cream cheese in the dairy department-but you can also use wild mushrooms and standard cream cheese.

Ingredients

- o 1 pound of rigatoni or similar pasta
- o 1 large package (12 oz.) of fresh mushrooms, cleaned and sliced
- o 1 large bag (10-12 oz.) of fresh baby spinach, washed well and stems removed
- o 1 cup walnut pieces
- o 3 tablespoons butter
- o 1 small container (8 oz.) mascarpone cheese
- o 1/2 cup freshly grated Parmesan cheese
- o Salt and fresh ground black pepper
- o 1/4 teaspoon freshly ground nutmeg or 1/2 teaspoon dried nutmeg.

Instructions

1. Place a big pot of water on to boil. (4 quarts or liters of pasta per pound)

2. While the water heats, carefully clean the mushrooms with a brush or a damp towel, cut off and slice the tough end of the stems. Do not run the mushrooms under water, as this makes them hard and chewy. To save time, look for fresh, pre-sliced mushrooms. In a large saucepan, melt the butter and sauté the mushrooms at medium low. Season gently with salt and pepper until they start exuding moisture. Continue to cook until the mushrooms are a dark golden brown and some of the fluid is drained.

3. Add the spinach and stir together until the spinach is just wilted.

4. Stir in the mascarpone cheese and 1/2 Parmesan cheese and combine well. Heat done. The mascarpone cheese starts to melt and thin out as it warms up a little. Spice with fresh nutmeg, black pepper salt and fresh-ground and turn the fire to low to stay dry.

5. Add 1 heaping tablespoon of salt while the water is at a rolling boil, and lower into the pasta. Stir gently to prevent sticking to the pasta. Cook until al dente (firm to bite) according to box instructions.

6. When the pasta is cooking, the walnuts softly toast on medium low heat in a hot, dry saucepan. Deposit back.

7. When the pasta is done, carefully reserve a 1/2 cup of the starchy pasta water and set aside. Drain the pasta and add it back into the hot pot, off the heat.

8. Add the mushroom and spinach sauce and toss everything together to combine. Add a splash of the reserved pasta water to smooth out the sauce to a silky consistency.

9. Plate the pasta and garnish with the toasted walnuts and the remainder of the Parmesan cheese. Serve immediately.

Recipe and Cooking Tips For Creamy Chicken Pot Pie

Chicken Pies are healthy things to enjoy. This Chicken Pot Pie Recipe is nothing more than the thing for a rich and tasty dinner dish. A great home cooked family dinner. The wine brings a beautiful taste to the filling of the pastry. You'll save time by using ready-made puff pastry.

You should prepare the entire thing in advance and then bake it before serving. A very smart idea, and time saver, is to make a double pie filling section and then freeze it in a pinch when you need a dinner. If you have learned the fundamentals, you should try tasteful combinations. Not exactly nice low-fat diet but good eaten with buttery mash and baby peas.

Some Chicken Pie Baking Tips

- o You can make the chicken pie ahead of time and bake it just before serving.
- o Make a double portion of the pie filling and then freeze it for when you need a meal in a hurry.
- o Always have a ready-made roll of puff pastry in the freezer for when you feel like pie.
- o Be sure to make a few small slits in the top of the pastry so that the steam can escape during the baking time.
- o Use left-over chicken or ready-cooked chicken if you want to save time.
- o Use vegetables in season as these will be cheaper and readily available.
- o Adjust the seasoning in the filling to suit your own taste.
- o Wine adds amazing depth to the flavor of the filling so if possible don't leave it out.
- o Chicken Pot Pie Recipe Ingredients
- o olive oil and butter, for frying
- o salt and milled pepper
- o 500g deboned chicken thighs, diced
- o 2 leeks, sliced
- o 2 celery sticks, sliced
- o 1 packet (250g) white or brown mushrooms, sliced
- o 2 cloves garlic, chopped

- o 2 Tbsp (30ml) thyme leaves
- o 1/2 cup (125ml) white wine
- o 1 cup (250ml) chicken stock
- o 1 tub (250ml) cream
- o 1 small packet (80g) baby spinach, blanched and chopped or frozen vegetable mix
- o 1 cup (250ml) fresh or frozen peas
- o 1 roll puff pastry, defrosted, divided into 4
- o 1 extra-large egg yolk, beaten

Cooking Instructions For Chicken and Mushroom Pot Pies

1.   Preheat oven to 220 C.

2.   Heat the oil and butter in pan and lightly saute the seasoned chicken until browned. Remove the cooked chicken from the pan and set aside.

3.   Fry the leeks, celery and mushrooms until soft but be careful not to brown too much. Add the chopped garlic and fry for another minute.

4.   Stir in the leaves of thyme, vinegar, chicken stock, milk and brown meat. Let this boil for about 25 minutes-the liquid will be decreased by half. Stir in wilted spinach and peas.

5. Filling the spoon into 4 ramekins / small pie dishes, filling each with pastry. Crimp edges with a fork and create a few slits in the pastry to allow steam to escape when they are baking from the chicken pies.

6. Place egg yolk on the tops of the pies and bake for 20 minutes or until the pastry has reached the wonderful golden color.

This Chicken Pot Pie serves 4 people.

RECIPES 4:   GREEK TURKEY BURGERS WITH TZATZIKI SAUCE-GYROS

Gyros, basically vertically grilled beef, tomatoes, onions, and tzatziki sauce, are commonly used as a lunch item worldwide. They're wonderful and all food classes are represented delivering the ideal midday meal.

What exactly is a Gyro?

The word for "shake" in itself derives from the Greek term and that is what it does. Food, usually pork, veal, or lamb, is piled in a cone and vertically broiled. A more traditional ingredient is chicken. The fat layers keep the rest of the meat tender while the sun makes the meat crisp too. The meat is cut from the cone very thinly and inserted inside a pita with potatoes, onions and tzatziki, a salad, garlic and cucumber sauce.

A more essential feature of the gyro is the spices. The beef is mixed in with paprika, oregano, salt, pepper and garlic. Everybody has their own secret. Others include parsley, allspice, or cumin, in addition to the other spices.

It is a traditional gyro. Nowadays you will find all kinds of fillings. In Greece it is also common to put fried potatoes in them and you can also find vegetarian varieties of falafel instead of meat. It is really just a sandwich then. Some can have pickled onions, cabbage, and mayonnaise as alternatives.

In Greece you can find the pita bread itself in plain, Cypriot, or Arabic. Simple is the most frequent, and of the three breaks the thickest. Cypriot is thinner and splits to make a pocket, while Arabic pita is crispier and flatter.

Origination

Unlike common opinion, gyros-pronounced "yee-ros "-did not originate in Greece, although the word was Greek in itself.

In reality Gyros is Turkish. Identified as a doner kebab in Turkey, they had been invented in the 19th century and shipped to Greece. They are close to shawarma which also begins in the Middle East.

The first gyro in the USA was built in Chicago in the mid-1960s. There's a bit of debate about who actually made the first gyro in Chicago, but there they were originally invented by a John Garlic, as told in a post published in the New York Times on July 14, 2009. No matter if they make it to the United States, the gyro remains an ever-popular staple of fast food and lunch, because they were not the first to catch on.

Build Your Own Tzatziki While you can place all kinds of sauces on the gyro, Greek tzatziki is usually the strongest. This spicy sauce has lots of garlic to taste, and the cucumber helps keep spices away from other ingredients in the soup.

Tzatziki's to make quick and easy. It tastes great as the spread of a burger, a veggie dip or even a salad dressing.

To make your own:

Put 1, 16 ounce Greek yogurt tub (the regular yogurt is too runny), half a finely chopped cucumber and two finely chopped cloves of garlic together. Season with white pepper and oil. For extra flavor some recommend adding chopped fresh dill and a bit of fresh lemon squeeze.

Gyros is one of the best fast-food options out there as long as you skip the fried potatoes, so they're a big step up from a two-dollar burger. They are packed full of flavor, and when prepared in the true manner, on a vertical rotisserie, there is nothing better.

Chicken Taco Soup

You need to have taco soup while dreaming of delicious snacks. It's perfect for heart-raising, and suitable when snowing outdoors. When you're out on holiday indoors it makes up for a perfect hot soup pot. The soup is a meal in itself. Making is pleasant, and perfect to have. What's stopping you from trying out the simple taco soup recipe? This is basically a simple recipe which is made from readily available ingredients. Your family is crying for more.

This is a recipe that has been tried and checked. Just follow it to get some delicious taco soup for your kin. A dutch oven, a slow cooker or even a stock bowl will do this.

It's easier to do this in a dutch oven, because there's no heat transfer in it. Cooking is hanging, and the soup is fine. Just seek it out and you will receive this recipe as a gift.

If you have fussy kids at home who don't have healthy food, so you've got to do it about them. The soup is delicious and healthy. The kids will press for more, so you will see them loving those healthy meals. The best thing about this is that it is as easy to cook this soup as consuming it is delicious.

You must first get all the ingredients needed to make this soup. These ingredients are easily available and it will not be difficult for you to get them. You will need the following.

- o   Red Beans (drained) - one can
- o   Ground beef - 1-1 1/2 lbs
- o   Black beans (drained) - one can
- o   Onion (chopped) - 1 small

- o Whole corn kernels (drained) - one can
- o Taco seasoning mix - 1 packet
- o Tomato Sauce - one can
- o Crushed tomatoes - one can
- o Diced Tomatoes - one can
- o Cheddar Cheese
- o Tortilla Chips
- o Chopped green onion
- o Sour cream

To cook this delicious hearty taco soup recipe you have to follow these steps.

1) In a stew pot or Dutch oven, you have to first cook the beef. Cook the beef with onion, salt and pepper. The beef has to brown all over. In case you need a hotter soup, you can even add cayenne pepper.

2) Add diced tomatoes, crushed tomatoes, taco seasoning, corn, beans and tomato sauce. Mix it very well.

3) Cook for about 2 hours, on low power. If you cook in a slow cooker the cooking will take 4-6 hours.

4) Serve with white sliced onions, sour cream, tortilla chips and cheddar cheese.

5. You may also use grilled chicken breasts instead of beef, if you wish.

When you're serving visitors with this broth, they'll ask you to recycle taco soups. The broth is delightful and stimulates the buds to taste. Anyone who has it would love this warm, spicy broth forever. And, if you're cooking the soup for your buddies or family, there'll definitely be more feedback coming. Since making this soap is fast and cheap you can use the formula as many times as you want.

RECIPES 5: WHITE CHEESE AND CHICKEN LASAGNA

This lasagna is perfect for any form of pot luck with a creamy white cheese sauce, pasta, and spinach. Good way to make your children eat spinach!

Ingredients

- o 9 lasagna noodles
- o 1/2 cup butter
- o 1 large white onion, chopped
- o 1 clove garlic, minced
- o 1/2 cup flour
- o 1 tsp salt
- o 2 cups chicken broth
- o 1 1/2 cups milk
- o 4 cups mozzarella cheese, shredded and divided
- o 1 cup Parmesan cheese, grated and divided
- o 1 tsp dried basil
- o 1 tsp dried oregano
- o 1/2 tsp pepper
- o 2 cups ricotta cheese
- o 2 cups cooked chicken breast, cubed
- o 2 (10 oz) packages frozen chopped spinach, thawed and drained
- o 1 tbsp fresh parsley, chopped
- o 1/4 cup grated Parmesan cheese
- o Directions
- o Preheat oven to 350 degrees.

o In a large pot boil lightly salted water. Add lasagna noodles and boil for 8 to 10 minutes. Drain. Rinse with cold water.

• In a large saucepan over medium heat, melt the butter. Sauté the onion and garlic in the butter until tender. Add the flour and salt. Mix well, and simmer until bubbly. Add the broth and milk to the pan, mix well, and boil. Stir constantly for 1 minute. Add 2 cups of the mozzarella cheese and 1/4 cup of the Parmesan cheese to the saucepan. Stir until well blended. Season with the basil, oregano, and pepper. Remove from heat. Set aside.

• Spread 1/3 of the sauce mixture in a 9×13 inch baking dish. Place 1/3 of the noodles, the ricotta, and the chicken in a layer over the sauce mixture.

• Place another layer of 1/3 of the noodles and then a layer of 1/3 of the sauce mixture.

• Place spinach and the remaining 2 cups of the mozzarella cheese and 1/2 cup of the Parmesan cheese in another layer.

• Lay the remaining noodles over the cheese, and spread remaining sauce evenly over noodles.

• Sprinkle with parsley and 1/4 cup Parmesan cheese.

• Bake 35 to 40 minutes. Let cool and rest before cutting and serving

Makes 12 servings.

Lasagna Recipe

Lasagna is a popular oven-baked pasta dish. The classic lasagna, if such a dish can be said to exist, is based on a meat and tomato ragu and a bechamel sauce. These are layered between sheets of pasta dough (two or three layers for a lasagna) in an oven dish, covered with cheese (usually parmesan or mozzarella) and baked in the oven for about half an hour.

Many lasagna variations exist. Vegetable lasagna, lasagna without bechamel, chicken lasagna, meatless cheese lasagna, lasagna without any sauce (just vegetables and/or meat) or even lasagna without the pasta.

When creating a lasagna, start with the main ingredient (ragu, vegetables, seafood, etc.), add a layer of bechamel, then one layer of pasta sheets and then the main ingredient again. Continue until the oven dish is full. End with a layer of pasta, spread some bechamel on top and sprinkle the cheese over it.

Some recipes call for the bechamel to be mixed through the ragu or tomato sauce, while others tell you to layer it between the pasta and the ragu. This seems to be based on personal preference and taste.

Besides sprinkling cheese on top of the lasagna, it's also a good idea to mix some through the bechamel sauce, to give the lasagna some cheese flavor throughout, instead of just on top. Turn the heat off under the bechamel sauce before adding the cheese, or the sauce will become rubbery.

There is a choice between home-made pasta and store-bought dried pasta when it comes to the pasta flour. Since dried pasta is made with only water and flour, and fresh home-made pasta normally contains eggs, a distinct difference in taste and texture is observed. Nevertheless, the biggest distinction comes from ease of use. Making pasta from scratch can be a long process which needs some practice in order to get it right.

Fresh pasta also needs to be precooked before assembling the lasagne. See the pasta page for a fresh pasta recipe.

Dried pasta is usually precooked, so it can be put in to the oven dish straight out of the packet.

In the US, pasta sheets generally have a curvy surface. Outside the US, they are almost always flat.

Here is a recipe for traditional lasagna.

Ingredients:

- o   2 tbsp olive oil
- o   1 large onion, finely chopped

- o 3 lbs Minced beef
- o 4 cloves of garlic, finely chopped or crushed
- o 1 can chopped plum tomatoes
- o 10-15 basil leaves, chopped or torn (or 1 tsp dried basil)
- o 1/2 tsp dried oregano
- o 5 crushed black peppercorns (or to taste)
- o 1 tsp sea salt (or to taste)
- o 1/2 tsp sugar
- o One pack of lasagna sheets
- o 1 1/2 pints Bechemel Sauce *

Finely grated parmesan

- o Bechemel Sauce:
- o 1/4 cup (4 Tablespoons) butter
- o 1/4 cup flour
- o 2 cups milk
- o Salt, white pepper, and nutmeg, as desired

Melt the butter in a sauce pan. Add the flour and whisk together over medium heat for 2-3 minutes. Do not allow to brown. Remove from heat and allow to cool nearly to room temperature.

Add hot milk and whisk to combine.

Stir in cinnamon, white pepper, and nutmeg, and heat until cooking is finished.

You should raise the sauce to a boil if desired; once the béchamel sauce has boiled down, lower the heat to low and simmer for about 45 minutes very slowly. Stir it with a whisk sometimes to avoid sticking to the rim. Do not have brown on the sauce. The longer the sauce is prepared, the better it is as the starch grains are fried and swelled

Preparation:

Heat the olive oil in a heavy base or non-stick pan over a medium-high heat. If the oil browns, turn the heat down.

Add the onion and fry until golden brown.

Increase heat to high and add the meat and garlic. Fry until brown. Minced/ground beef takes some time to cook well. Fry until there is little moisture left in the pan. If necessary, spoon out any excess fat.

Add the tomatoes, cover the pan and lower the heat and simmer for 20 minutes. Meanwhile, prepare the bechemel sauce.

Pre-heat the oven to 375 f.

Mix the basil, oregano, salt & pepper in to the ragu.

Place a thin layer of ragu in the base of the ovenproof dish and cover with a single layer of pasta sheets. Spread a layer of bechemel sauce over the pasta. Repeat this until you run out of meat, making sure that you have enough bechemel sauce left to cover the top layer of pasta.

Sprinkle the grated parmesan over the top.

Place the dish in the oven on the top shelf and cook for about 45 minutes, or until the top is lightly browned and the sauce is bubbling.

Secrets to Perfect White Sauce and How to Use It

I call these tips secrets because I never find them in cook books, but they are so simple. I've used white sauces frequently since I was a newlywed and learned how versatile they are. Along the way, I figured out some things that just make a better sauce, and a trick or two that save about half the work, and give it a smoother, silkier texture.

Basic white sauce is great to throw together as a binder for lots of dishes, and invaluable for casseroles. Get the basic recipe down and you can alter it by adding herbs and spices, cheese, wine or whatever to fit what you're making. I use the same basic recipe for Italian, Mexican or plain old American. It all depends on what you add.

The three most common problems with white sauce are a pasty flavor, the time you have to stand over the pot slowly adding the liquid, and those icky lumps.

- To avoid a floury, pasty taste, brown the flour in the butter until it just begins to turn golden. Watch out, though, it can scorch and that's gross. If it does, throw it out and start over. Trust me; it's better than serving a disgusting casserole or cheese sauce. It's best to keep the temperature at medium or lower.

- My next tip actually takes care of both the time issue and the lumps. To save a few minutes and avoid little lumps, heat the liquid in a separate pot or the microwave while you work with the butter and flour mixture. Pour the hot liquid into the golden flour mixture all at once, blending quickly with a wire whisk. You can step away from it for a couple minutes at a time to work on other parts of the meal, and just come back and whisk it again. Just don't leave it too long or it will scorch. Make sure you whisk everything off the bottom each time you come back to stir it. This is the technique that really thrilled me to discover, because it's almost impossible to end up with lumpy sauce this way.

Basic White Sauce

Ingredients

- o 1 1/2 c milk
- o 3/4 c broth
- o 2 Tb butter
- o 1/2 small onion, diced
- o 3 cloves garlic, smashed, skins removed, and diced
- o 1/4 tsp coarse salt, a few grinds fresh pepper

- 1/4 c flour
- Fresh nutmeg (my secret ingredient)

Preparation

1) Heat milk and broth together in a small pot (or microwave in a bowl)
2) Heat large pot or saute pan over medium high, add butter, turn down to medium or medium low, let melt
3) Add onion and garlic to the melted butter, season with salt and a few grinds of pepper, saute until onion is softened
4) Whisk flour into butter, onion and garlic until just golden
5) Pour in hot liquid all at once; whisk vigorously until well blended and smooth
6) Stir occasionally until sauce begins to thicken
7) Add a couple gratings of fresh ground nutmeg
8) Remove from heat when thickened, it will continue to thicken as it cools
9) Variations:
10) Add about 1 cup of salsa and 1/2 cup cheese and heat through for a great Mexican white sauce. This one is awesome for chicken tacos and burritos
11) Replace the 1/2 cup of broth with wine, but add the wine to the flour butter mixture, letting it boil off and thicken
12) Season with more garlic, add Italian seasonings and 1/2 cup of Parmesan cheese for an Italian sauce. For a different take on lasagna, replace the ricotta cheese with the Parmesan sauce.
13) In a separate skillet, saute broccoli or asparagus and cubed chicken or beef. Pour the sauce over and stir to incorporate. Serve over mashed or baked potatoes,

noodles, or rice, etc. Be sure to season the meat and veggies with salt, pepper and whatever else you like, or the overall flavor will be too bland. You can also add some grated cheese. Of course, use whatever vegetable and meat sounds good to you.

14) Add 1/4 cup of Dijon mustard for mustard gravy for roast, meatloaf, chicken breasts or potatoes.

15) Add drained diced tomatoes and some Worcestershire sauce for another twist on gravy.

16) For cheese sauce: at the start of the cooking, add a little more of either the broth or milk (about 1/4 cup or so). The cheese thickens it, even if it's still deep you end up with a mass of cheese instead of cheese sauce! Add 1/2 to 1cup of your choice of cheese, (stronger cheeses hold more spice in the sauce) only before they are ready to use, extract from heat and mix gently to apply.

An extra suggestion on cheese sauces: Don't run over. If it's overcooked or over-stirred it does weird things to the texture.

Yeah, you have it. A great basis for plenty of tasty dishes to please your family, your friends or even yourself!

RECIPES 6:   GARLIC CHEESY BREAD

Spaghetti, pasta, pizza and so on, are all incomplete when eaten with spicy garlic bread. The advantage of a recipe for bread from garlic cheese is that you can add your own slight twist. About any meal you prepare in the kitchen goes along with these. Garlic cheese breads are often eaten as a snack with tea and snacks, and it is a favorite of kids when eaten as garlic bread sticks.

Here is a simple recipe for bread from garlic cheese with little twists:

Tangy garlic cheese bread

Ingredients

Bread (any kid you like). You can use a loaf or separate slices.

1-2 heads of garlic (depending on your taste). If you are serving as a side dish use more garlic but if serving as a snack use less amount of garlic Chives and parsley chopped

1-2 sticks of butter

Zest of lemon

Cajun spice seasoning - 2 tablespoon

1 cup of grated cheese

Method

In a cup, brown the garlic and add milk, chives, parsley, lemon zest, butter and cajun seasoning. Let it rest for a bit until all the flavors blend. Take the slices of bread and scatter the mix onto the slices. If you are in the middle taking a loaf slip and adding the blend to form a sandwich. Bake the bread for 15 minutes in a preheated 200 C oven. Serve moist.

Soft garlic cheese bread

Ingredients

Bread of your choice Different types of cheeses mixed together -1 cup (parmesan, feta etc.)

Butter -2 sticks

Garlic cloves -15 or 20 Garlic

salt - 1 tablespoon

Herbs of your choice -1 teaspoon

Milk -1 teaspoon

Method

Melt the butter in a microwave and the milk together. Let the mixture cool down, then add the cheese, the crushed garlic, the oil, the herbs. To get a creamy butter like consistency mix well and bring it into a blender. Apply the mixture to slices of bread. Cover the slices of bread in silver foil and seal them securely. Even some extra cheese you can add on the slices. Preheat the oven at 220, and roast for 15-20 minutes the silver foil wrapped in sugar. Serve moist.

You can also make ham, chicken, potato grilled sandwiches with a fluffy garlic bread to enjoy for lunch the next day. Serve the bread with a cucumber dip or salsa and share your evening tea's enhanced flavor. Replace regular butter with low-fat butter and cheese with low-fat cheese for those who are diet conscious.

Monkey Bread-Sweet and Savory

Below are two Monkey Bread tips, a type of pull-apart pizza. Such breads are made by cutting dough into pieces, filling them with seasonings and bringing together the seasoned pieces before baking. We use refrigerated biscuit dough store-purchased here. The soft monkey bread includes cinnamon, sugar, and almonds, while the garlic and cheese are on the savory side.

Usually I bake these in a loaf pan, but you can use a Bundt pan or two loaf pans to double the recipe. When it comes to buying the biscuit dough, don't get the kind with layers. Pillsbury Grands! is probably the most widely used, but a store brand version would work too. I once accidentally got the kind with dots of butter throughout the dough, and the resulting bread was extra rich and decadent.

There are two ways of bringing together such breads. One way: in molten butter, coat the bits of dough, cover them in the seasonings and then layer them in the oven. Another way: put the seasonings in a plastic bag, place the bits of dough in the bag and shake, bring the bread together and add the melted butter over the end.

Cinnamon-Sugar Monkey Bread

- one 16.5 oz can of refrigerated biscuits
- 1 stick of butter, melted (1/2 cup)
- 1 tablespoon ground cinnamon
- 3/4 cup granulated sugar
- 1/2 cup pecans (optional)

Oven preheat to 350 degrees Fahrenheit. Grease the frying pan. Stir in sugar and cinnamon. Break the biscuits (4 parts each) into halves. Dip each slice into butter, then sprinkle with cinnamon sugar. Place the coated pieces in the saucepan. Sprinkle pecans between layers if desired. Pour over the prepared egg, the remaining butter and cinnamon-sugar. Bake for 40 minutes or when forced down, before the bread rises or springs down. Invert the bread onto a plate after the baking is done: put a plate on top of the loaf tin, turn it upside down and let the bread fall out. Take the pieces out to feed.

Cheesy-Garlic Monkey Bread

- o One 16.5 oz can of refrigerated biscuits
- o Half a stick of butter, melted (1/4 cup)
- o 3 cloves garlic, minced
- o 3/4 cup grated Parmesan
- o 1 teaspoon thyme or other herb of your choice

350 degrees Fahrenheit, preheat the oven. Grease the frying pan. Combine the garlic, parmesan and thyme, and dump the mixture into a plastic container. Break the biscuits into pieces, then drop the bits of dough into the plastic container. Cover the bag and shake with garlic-Parmesan mixture to coat the bits. Take the dough out of the container and place it in the greased saucepan. Pour the melted butter over the bread and scatter over the top of the remaining garlic-Parmesan combination. Bake for 20 minutes or more, before the bread is full. Invert the oven, so that the bread sits on a plate upside down. Step back to eat.

Garlic Cheese Biscuits

Eating a restaurant is one of the most challenging things to do while dining gluten free. Usually we're left with few options including a beef without sauce, a salad and plain vegetables. As gratifying as it is to be forced to eat at a gluten-restricted restaurant, it's almost shameful to sit down and watch your wheat eating mates devour the rolls, bread or biscuits! My mind is not going to stop dreaming about the delicious brown bread or the rolls of mouth-watering garlic cheese and I have to make some when I get home!

If your gluten-free restaurant experience leaves you starving for food, try my much sought after, simple recipe for these soft, crispy, buttered garlic biscuits!

You will need a food processor. There are many adaptations of this recipe on the Internet.

It is my version of brown rice for nutritious benefit as the principal flour ingredient. If you've never baked gluten free, you'll have to make a run to the flours and zanthan gum natural food store (made from corn and used in other foods like ice cream, sauces, and salad dressings). On the pricey side, your initial purchase might sound a little costly but you will make so much more than just one batch of these tasty biscuits. This flour blend can be used to make lots of gluten free cookies and breads! You should consider it a lot greater choice than attempting to fulfill your needs for gluten-free bread with the pre-made variants on the shelves which come with an expensive price and a taste reminiscent of buttered cardboard!

Gluten Free Garlic Cheese Biscuits

- ○ ½ cup potato starch
- ○ ¾ cup brown rice flour
- ○ 1 ¾ teaspoons Xanthan Gum
- ○ 1 tbsp baking powder
- ○ ¼ tsp baking soda
- ○ ½ tsp salt
- ○ 1 tbsp sugar
- ○ 1/3 cup cold butter cut into 1/4 inch cubes (or favorite margarine substitute)
- ○ ¾ cup buttermilk (or substitute by adding 1 tbsp white vinegar to ¾ cup regular milk and let sit 5 mins)
- ○ 1/2 cup shredded cheddar cheese
- ○ ¼ cup butter (or favorite substitute)
- ○ ¼ tsp garlic powder

While oven is preheating at 375 degrees F, spray a cookie sheet or pizza pan with cooking spray.

Using a regular blade on your food processor, pulse together the potato starch, brown rice flour, Xanthan Gum, baking powder, baking soda, salt and sugar; eight pulses, one second each.

Place butter pieces over the mixture and pulse processor 15 pulses or until mixture resembles large crumbs.

Pour buttermilk or substitute over the mixture. Pulse eight times or until dough rolls into a soft ball.

Add shredded cheddar cheese. Pulse 3 times or until cheese is distributed.

Drop dough onto sheet by lightly scooping small handfuls and gently dropping into a ball shape, (these won't be perfectly round, they are drop style biscuits).

Bake 10 - 12 minutes or until lightly browned.

As biscuits are baking melt ¼ cup butter and mix in garlic powder.

Brush butter and garlic powder mixture on tops of all biscuits.

Makes 6 - 8 biscuits.

Enjoy while warm and satisfy your soft biscuit craving!

Cheesy Chicken Lasagna

My families love of lasagna and cheese lead me to this recipe. The more cheese the better as far as they are concerned. It was a real hit at our bible studies brunch, and I have taken it to several other functions and each time several people want the recipe. So I thought I would share it with the world.

I have served it with a salad and a good crusty bread, and with vegetables and the bread. The grandkids really love it, more so than regular lasagna. I think it is the cheese, I could put cheese on just about anything and they would love it. If your looking for a tasty way to switch up you lasagna, give this recipe a try.

What you will need:

- 1 (10.75-oz.) can condensed cream of chicken soup
- 1 (10.75-oz.) can condensed cream of mushroom soup
- 1 cup chicken broth
- 1/2 tsp. garlic powder
- 6 lasagna noodles, cooked and drained
- 4 cups chopped cooked chicken breast
- 3 cups shredded mild Cheddar cheese
- 1-1/2 cups shredded low-moisture part-skim mozzarella cheese

The first thing to do is to preheat your oven to 350 degrees. Next, in a large bowl whisk together the chicken soup, mushroom soup, broth and garlic powder; set aside.

Using a rectangle 2-quart baking dish, layer half the lasagna noodles, half the chicken, half the soup mixture and half the Cheddar cheese. Repeat the layers and top with the mozzarella cheese.

Bake, open, for 35 minutes, or until the sides are bubbly heated clean. Only let it stand before serving for 10 minutes. This will allow the lasagna to firm up a little before you cut in it. The parts of the cut would be much better served if allowed to stand before cutting.

The estimated preparation time for this lasagna is about 15 minutes, and the estimated cooking time is about 35 minutes. They're going to eat 8. This really simple, quick and cheesy recipe is a favorite crowd, hope you will enjoy it just as much as my family!

Cheesy Spanish Rice Recipe

Once you've learned to love rice and admire the multiple variables, this recipe is sure to make you excited to try it. It's very fast and it's simple, you do need to know that's very tasty. Keep a quick look at the steps ahead and be prepared to enjoy this rice at dinner time in your house.

You will need:

- o Ground beef (1/2 pound)
- o Green Pepper (1 large, diced)
- o Onion (1/2 cup, chopped)
- o White rice (2 cups, cooked)
- o Garlic (1 clove, minced)
- o Tomato soup (1 can or 10.75 ounce undiluted)

- o Cheese food (4 ounces, cubed)
- o Chili powder (1 teaspoon)
- o Salt (1/4 teaspoon)
- o Pepper (1/4 teaspoon)

How to do it:

Take a big skillet and cook the beef, green pepper, onion and garlic in here, do all this over medium heat and once the meat is no longer white, then rinse the mixture and then add the pasta, vinegar, chili powder, add the salt and pepper. You'll need to cook this before the cheese is melted and then pass most of the mix to a 3-cup baking platter. When you have the cover and bake the mixture for about 35 minutes at 350o-Fahrenheit degrees. Now that you've done this you can take it out of the oven and enjoy it aside with a little toast, or maybe with a cooling soda. It's quite easy and by adding some fresh parsley you can also give it a more trendy look top.

RECIPES 7: PESTO CHICKEN PASTA BAKE-ITALIAN RECIPE SUN-DRIED TOMATO PESTO WITH CHICKEN

As a main course:

Sun-dried tomato pesto is amazing. I sometimes eat it with the fresh noodles for lunch. If you delete the chicken from the recycle below, the pesto can be used as a primo course on noodles (first), as spreads on crostini (toasted thin bread), fish, etc. I attached the chicken to make it a main course. Also you can swap the chicken with Italian sausage (about 6 links, cut) for a main course.

Ingredients (5 servings):

- o 1 pound - fresh pasta (penne if you can find it fresh)
- o 3 - skinless, boneless chicken breasts
- o 2 bottles (7 ounces each) - sun-dried tomatoes, oil drained
- o 5 ounces - Parmesan cheese
- o 1/4 cup - fresh basil (washed and packed in the cup)
- o 3 tablespoons - pine nuts

- 6 cloves - garlic
- 3/4 cup - extra virgin olive oil
- Salt and pepper to taste

Preparation:

Preheat oven to 350 F. In the meantime, boil a couple of quarters of water in a salted pot and prepare the penne (fresh pasta will only take a few minutes). While waiting for the water to boil, the chicken breasts are rinsed and any fat removed. Place in a baking dish and cook in the oven for about 30 to 40 minutes, until brown and well baked. Switch off the oven until the breasts are done but do not disconnect until the pasta has been baked.

In a food processor, add the sun-dried tomatoes, Parmesan cheese, basil, pine nuts, garlic and olive oil and blend until fully combined (can be cooled for up to two weeks, covered).

When the pasta is finished, set aside 1/2 cup water from the boiling pot, and then drain the pasta well. Place the pasta back into the cooking pot, add the sun-dried tomato pesto and mix well.

Remove the chicken from the oven and dice. Add the chicken along with salt and pepper and the 1/2 cup pasta water. Cook on medium high heat while mixing until it is hot enough to serve.

Italian Recipe-Basil Pesto

Origins: Basil pesto comes from the northern Italian City of Genoa (pesto alla genovese). Pesto in Italian is derived from a word which means beating or crushing. The food was obviously called before they had food processors.

Can you see all the ingredients shredding together? A basil cheese spread as far back as Roman times is listed but it was the Genovese who first mixed all the traditional ingredients. It was not until the 1940s (probably because of World War II) that basil pesto started to be mentioned in newspapers. And it did not become a popular dish in America until the 1980s and 1990s. I call it a "triple crown" recipe - easy to make, healthy, and delicious. In a later article, I will show you how to make sundried tomato pesto also.

Other uses: I might also add that although my recipe calls for the basil pesto to be added to pasta, you can use it on baked potatoes, spread over crostini (thinly-sliced toasted bread), or you can use it to season fish and chicken dishes.

Ingredients (5 servings):

- o   2 cups (about 5 ounces) - fresh basil, pressed or packed (approximately - i.e., take the basil leaves and press them into a cup)
- o   3 cloves - garlic
- o   1/4 cup - pine nuts
- o   4 ounces - parmesan, grated
- o   1/2 cup - extra virgin olive oil
- o   1/2 teaspoon - salt
- o   Pepper to taste
- o   1 pound - fresh pasta (linguine or fettuccine)

Preparation:

Rinse the basil leaves and place them in a food processor along with the garlic, pine nuts, parmesan cheese, and olive oil and blend until well mixed

Add pepper to taste and mix.

Meanwhile, cook the pasta in a few quarts of water (if it is fresh pasta it should only take a few minutes). Drain the pasta and place back in the pot. Add the basil pesto and mix well. Serve hot.

Pasta Recipe Ideas Every Mother Should Know

Kids are mostly picky eater and they like to eat sweet and junks instead of having something healthy and appetizing. It's actually a role of a mother that how she handles the situation and make her kid eat everything which is cooked for that day. However, at times kids should get to eat something of their wish, something which they like to eat but without forgetting the healthy part.

Just because they are demanding for a quick bite of a junk food doesn't mean you can't alter a food which is not just taste like their favorite fast foods but healthy too. If we check universally, after chocolates, sweets and ice creams kids like pasta and pizza the most. Italian recipes are known for its subtle flavors which are very much appreciated by kids. Mostly kids avoid spicy and hot food and prefer nice creamy, cheesy recipes. So in today's post, we will discuss the top 10 pasta recipes which are kid's friendly, easy to make and moreover healthy.

1. Country Chicken Noodle Soup: Chicken noodle soups are one of the simplest recipe that you can make for your kids and the best thing about this soup is you can try different alternatives with different vegetables and types of pasta. It's a flavorsome recipe with chicken, veggies and whole grain pasta.

2. Gluten-free Pasta (Zucchini Spaghetti with Spinach and Pesto): This recipe is for this kids who are gluten sensitive. This recipe is delightful recipe which is not just healthy for kids but delectable too even after adding spinach. To make the pasta grate the fresh zucchini and toss it with vibrant green cashew and spinach pesto.

3. Mac and Cheese: It's a recipe which is not just a favorite of our kids but also love by adults. This cheesy, creamy pasta recipe is although full of cheese but cheese is good for body if taken in moderate. And as it is said, it's okay to indulge at times to give some treats and perks.

4. Rainbow Pasta: As the name suggest, it is a colorful pasta recipe which kids love to eat. In the kids psychology it's been proved that kids attracts to colorful

things, so if you can add some beautiful color in their food, then we are sure they will never skip their meals.

5. Pasta salad: Another classic recipe loved by all. Since its summer, kids love something cold and refreshing and pasta salad is the solution to this problem. Pasta salad is full of vegetables and if you are making it with chicken then it is a complete meal.

6. Chicken Lo Mein: This is an Asian inspired pasta recipe which is not just tasty and delicious but easy to make too. It just got simple steps and at the end you will get this amazing kid's approved recipe within 30 minutes. Feel free to add more veggies if you feel like.

7. Baked Pasta: A fuss free recipe which is loved by kids. Simply mix the ingredients and cheese and let it bake at 350 degree F. Cheddar cheese, tomatoes, penne pasta, broccoli, peas or whatever you want to add. Simply mix all the ingredients in the boiled pasta and let it bake till the cheese melts.

8. Lasagna: Another classic pasta recipe which is universally accepted. Its super yummy and kids love the layer of goodness in this recipe. Add different mashed vegetables, minced meat and another healthy ingredients to make this recipe healthy and nourishing. Add zucchini and pumpkin to add the extra flavor and taste.

9. Creamy Tomato Pasta: A super quick simple recipe made from fresh or sun-dried tomato and cheddar

cheese. Flavors are refreshing and delicious and it's really simple to make. Simple make a puree of tomatoes, add cheese of your choice and cook pasta by adding fresh herbs and seasoning.

10. Chicken Penne: Did you know penne is Vitamin A-rich? For full benefits often recommend whole grain pasta. It's a hearty recipe with Mexican flavors, and preparing for a busy weekend as well is very fast.

Above are accepted pasta recipes for best boy. All the recipes are not just easy to make but are really delicious. And if you have a special recipe for your kid that you'd love to share, please comment below. This way more moms will interact and thoroughly share their insights and recipes. Good gourmet food!

RECIPES 8:   SLOW-COOKER ORANGE CHICKEN-BARBECUED CHICKEN WITH TANGY ORANGE SAUCE

You crave for the BBQ occasionally. You want so much barbecue you can smell it and taste it. The sort of barbecue you want depends on where you have been spending your youth and where you are now living. The so-called "sides" differ even depending on the venue.

Hormel Foods has a barbecue sauce map on their web site. Barbecue developed in Virginia and North Carolina in the late 18th century, the site says, and began as a vinegar dipping sauce for pork.

Time passed and more ingredients were added to the sauce. People in North Carolina like a sweet, vinegar-based sauce. The folks in South Carolina add mustard to their recipe. If you grew up in the Smoky Mountains you like sauce made with tomatoes, ketchup, and vinegar.

Florida residents are adding lemon and lime juice to their sauce, as you would expect. Residents of Alabama like a sweet sauce while residents of Kentucky like their deep one. Words to define Texas barbecue are hot and spicy.

Memphis people use molasses to flavor their tomato flavored sauce.

Like me, midwesteners love a thick sauce, based on tomatoes. For years I was cooking my barbecue sauce up from scratch. The recipe had several ingredients, molasses included, and it took half an hour to make. So, I got a faster version of the recipe. I add molasses when I cook pork but then I use orange marmalade when I cook chicken. In five minutes, you can make the sauce, and enjoy the smell for hours. Serve barbecue chicken with coleslawed rice and fruit. Double the recipe while you're teen cooking.

INGREDIENTS

- o 2 1/2 pounds skinless chicken breasts
- o 1 tablespoon extra light olive oil
- o 1 3/4 cups barbecue sauce (lowest sugar/salt content you can find)
- o 1 cup fresh orange juice
- o 1/2 cup sugar-free orange marmalade
- o 1 tablespoon orange zest, diced
- o 2 green onions, white and green parts, chopped

METHOD

Cover with olive oil on a well seasoned cast iron skillet. Cut in two long strips of each chicken breast. Saute the stripes over medium to high heat until they tend to tan. Switch the strips of chicken to slow cooker.

Use paper towels to clean any residual oil from skillet. Barbecue sauce, orange juice, marmalade, orange zest, and green onions are mixed into the same pan. Heat the sauce and pour over the chicken until it begins to simmer. Cover and simmer for about 6 hours at low. Requires 5–6 pieces.

Chicken Noodle Soup

Chicken Noodle Soup is one of my specialties. The formula I use is special in the way I do it every time. It is my own idea, one of those tests that falls from my brain, never written down. I'll put this and that together, as with the rest of my recipes; a few of this and a few shakes of that. When I use a recycle, I never totally obey it the way it is printed.

This is a recipe is for a slow cooker, but a large stock pan can be substituted. Adjust the seasoning to your taste.

- o 3 1/2 to 4 lbs. frying chicken
- o 1 large onion (or 2 medium) - diced
- o 3 carrots, sliced
- o 3 celery stalks, sliced
- o 1 tsp. salt
- o 1/2 tsp. pepper

- o 2 tsp. lemon pepper
- o 1 tsp. basil
- o 1/2 tsp. thyme
- o 2 tsp. parsley flakes (crushed)
- o 1/2 tsp sage
- o 2 tsp. beef bouillon (or 2 cubes)
- o 2 tsp chicken bouillon (or 2 cubes)
- o 1 1/2 to 2 c. 100% orange juice
- o 2 1/2 to 3 c. egg noodles
- o 5 c. of water
- o 1 c. of water for bouillon

Thoroughly wash the chicken, strip off the skin and trim out any extra fat. Put chicken with 5 cups of water (or enough to cover meat) in slow cooker. Take the Slow Cooker instructions. In most cases fire up to boil at 300 degrees, then simmer for 3 to 4 hours. When the meat comes off the bone, chicken is cooked.

Cut the vegetables, and set aside at the time you prepare the chicken.

Taking it out of the cooker until the chicken is cooked, debon the chicken and cut it into pieces. Strain the broth into a strainer, with any fragile bones. (You can also strain it through cheesecloth to trap some of the grease. The fat can also be removed by chilling the broth overnight and skimming off the layer of fat from the top.)

Add back all of the broth to the slow cooker. Place the bouillon in the cup of hot water and mix until dissolved. Add the bouillon mixture and the orange juice to the slow cooker. Combine the chicken, vegetables and spices to the slow cooker. Heat the soup to boil and then simmer for at least an hour or until vegetables are tender.

Cook the egg noodles according to the directions, and then add to the pot. Cook another 30 minutes.

Makes about 4 1/2 quarts

Serves 10 (or 4 very hungry people)

Added notes:

Soup can be placed in smaller containers for the freezer. Soup can be frozen for several months.

Healthy Lentil Stew For Slow Cooker Recipe

If you have not tried lentils in your new plan of healthy eating, crock pot stew is a good place to begin. Lentils readily absorb the flavors around them. They are quick and easy to prepare, always available, and as you will see, filled with healthy nutrients.

Lentils provide six minerals, two B vitamins, and protein. They supply generous amounts of folate and magnesium and iron. Lentils are a good cholesterol-lowering legume;

rich in fiber and nutrients, and no fat. All these nutrients go far in helping manage blood-sugar levels.

Lentils are harvested in many colors; choose brown or green ones to hold shape in dishes requiring long cooking times. Yellow, red, or orange varieties tend to soften easier and get mushy when cooked too long. For that reason, colored varieties lend themselves well to salads and vegetable dishes. The color does not seem to vary the subtle nutty flavor

Unlike beans, lentils do not need pre-soaking. They do, however, need washed thoroughly and checked carefully for small stones or debris. Because they are so small, spread them out evenly on a lightly colored plate to sort. Then wash them in a sieve.

If you are planning to cook lentils on the stove top, add three cups of water to each cup of lentils. Follow the directions on the bag and check often to get the needed firmness.

For our Crock Pot recipe, we will use raw, washed lentils.

- o Lentil Stew
- o 3 cups lentils (1 lb.)
- o 3 cups water
- o 1 can diced tomatoes with liquid
- o 1 can chicken broth

Chop and add the following vegetables: 4 stalks celery, 1 large onion, 1 green bell pepper, 1 large carrot, and 2 cloves garlic.

Add ¼ tsp black pepper and 1 tsp dried marjoram leaves.

Combine above ingredients and cook covered on Low 8 to 9 hours.

Stir in 2 Tablespoons of cider vinegar and 2 tablespoons of olive oil after cooking (adjust as per taste).

Lentil stew is well eaten over rice or couscous, and will hold for up to one week in the refrigerator. The stew can be stored in an airtight jar and preserved for up to three months.

This is a good stew to freeze in small portions for those nights when you are too tired to cook and tend to grab a less nutritious snack.

Soon you will be finding lentils a favorite item to stock in your cabinets. The variety of uses is endless; cold in salads and vegetable dishes; added to casseroles and main dishes, and tossed into soups and chilis.

You will soon find the added nutrition and protein lentils provide will give you a real perk-me-up on those tiring evenings when you are done and your day isn't! Personally, I am wondering where have they been all my life?

RECIPES 9: BERRY BANANA SMOOTHIE- ACAI BERRY DIET SMOOTHIES

Acai berry diet smoothies are super tasty and simple to produce. This Brazilian super fruit was suggested by fitness enthusiasts, scientific professionals and celebrities alike. The Acai berry diet is a food high in antioxidants, vitamins, minerals, healthy fatty acids and all kinds of other important nutrients necessary for your longevity and good health.

A smoothie is one of the best supplements you can make on this fruit. This will help you detoxify your body and weight loss, which are among the strongest benefits behind Acai. This fruit is extremely rich in the right kind of fibers, so it is recommended for the morning and midday when you have time to work off the carbohydrates. Here is the best way to make a delicious smoothie that you will love, and benefit from.

Ingredients: Acai berry powder or concentrate, single banana, milk (or, if you want to, sub-soy milk), strawberry frozen yogurt and a blender.

Preparation: Pick your Acai berry juice or paste, and pour into your blender a standard serving amount. Before the water, pour a cup of normal milk or soy milk in. When appropriate use low fat or non-fat types. Slice the banana into chunks then drop it in for a smooth texture. Finally add half a cup of raspberry ice yogurt, subdue if necessary for a low fat variety. Blend for 20 to 30 seconds, and enjoy!

Each morning you should have a smoothie for breakfast and each day you kick start your Acai berry diet the right way!

Mango Lassi, Berry Banana Smoothie, and Chai

Mango Lassi

Mangoes contain phenols that give the capacity to be antioxidant and anticancer. They're also rich in magnesium, perfect for pregnant women and anemia sufferers. Digestive mangoes benefit because they are rich in antioxidants and low in carbohydrates. Good for diabetics, and anybody battling kidney disease, as well as a decent source of vitamin A, E and selenium.

- o 1 Large mango, or 1 Cup of mango chunks
- o 1 Cup of plain yogurt
- o 1/2 Cup of milk
- o 1/4 Cup of Odwalla's MangoTango
- o 1/4 Cup crushed Ice
- o 2 teaspoons of honey
- o If you like a spicey Lassi (1/2 teaspoon of cardamom)

Blend all together in a blender or food processor.

Berry Banana Smoothie

The Berry Banana Smoothie is rich with potassium and vitamin C. This recipe also has yogurt in it, that gives it natural probiotics, essential for digestion. Berry Smoothies give you more fiber and nutrients than regular juices, helping you to stay properly hydrated, while supporting your immune system. You can also substitute red, yellow raspberries or even blue berries. I've tried grapes, don't go there, it's yucky.

- 1 Banana
- 8 Strawberries
- 10 black berries
- 1/2 Cup vanilla yogurt
- 1/2 Cup Odwalla's Orange Juice
- Blend and serve!

Chai

Health benefits of chai are that you aren't drinking coffee. There's roughly 3 times more caffeine in comparing one cup of coffee to one cup Chai. All of the different spices, cinnamon, cardamom, nutmeg, cloves, ginger, all have tremendous antioxidant powers, that have proven to be very beneficial to long term health. All of these spices are supportive to the repair of organs in the body.

- 3 Cups of Water
- Black Tea (6 tea bags) or 5 tablespoons of black loose tea
- 2 teaspoon of finely chopped fresh ginger root
- 3 cinnamon sticks (or 1 teaspoon of powdered cinnamon)
- 1 teaspoon of cardamom
- 1 teaspoon of nutmeg
- 1/4 teaspoon of cloves
- 1 1/2 teaspoons of vanilla extract
- 1 Tablespoon of honey (less if you don't like it sweet)
- Bring All ingredients to a boil in a small sauce pan, and boil for 2 min.
- Then Add: 1/2 Cup of Half&Half
- 1/2 Cup of 2% Milk

Serve hot, or over ice. Add Whip cream on top!

These are great afternoon snacks for everyone, although I would hold off on giving Chai to children, as it still contains more caffeine than they need. I hope you enjoy these recipes, and look forward to hearing your comments on them.

Banana Smoothies Recipe

Who doesn't enjoy a smoothie on a hot day, whether you're relaxing on the deck or hurrying to school or work? Versatile, delicious, made in a flash - and full of nutrients; recipes for banana smoothies. Children love them and whipping a couple of them up before school will make sure they have a nutritious breakfast to get them through the day.

Banana smoothies recipe? For breakfast? Why not? Bananas contain tryptophan - a protein which the body converts into serotonin. And serotonin is a natural hormone which helps to regulate mood; that's the ingredient in most anti-depression medications. And if you're taking diuretics, certain ones can deplete the body's reserves of potassium - two bananas a day will correct that. Bananas also contain iron as well as those essential trace elements and most vitamins too. They possess a natural antacid which helps digestion, colitis, diarrhea and constipation and, as the commercial says - it's the "foodiest" fruit of all.

The healthiest way to eat bananas is when the skin has turned almost black. Agreed, they don't look so appetizing, but all their properties are at their maximum at that point - just peel them and toss them in the blender. And did you know that you can freeze bananas - peel them, cut them in half, package and freeze. They replace the ice in your banana smoothies recipe, keeping it cold and putting less of a load on your blender. Most people use milk to make smoothies, but you can use soy milk, ice-cream, rice milk, chocolate milk and perhaps a drizzle of honey or maple syrup for sweetness. You can buy frozen berries out of season and add a handful to your own recipes for banana smoothies.

Here's one your children will love - peanut butter with your own banana smoothies recipe and this is enough for two. Two frozen bananas, ten ounces of milk (try almond milk) and two tablespoons of peanut butter. Whirl them all together in the blender and hey presto.

Fresh strawberries added to your own recipes for banana smoothies are delectable in fresh berry season. This amount is for one adult - one whole banana, a cup of sliced fresh strawberries and eight ounces of cold milk (try soy milk here). Blend on medium speed, taste and add more milk if it's too thick. Try blueberries or raspberries in your recipes for banana smoothies - delicious. Take your frothy creation out on the deck and enjoy watching the birds feed their chicks.

So, bananas and milk, or a substitute for milk, are your main ingredients for your banana smoothies recipe. Add whatever fruits or juices you want, merrily blend it all together and know that even if it sounds disgusting, it's not a "guilt food;" you're eating something that's packed with antioxidants, tastes great, elevates your mood-and it's breakfast going, so you can take it to work in your cup.

All correct. Yet. For two men, this is one of those rare Banana smoothies recipes. Two ripe bananas, two scoops of vanilla ice cream (the right stuff), a quarter teaspoon of coffee, eight ounces of whole milk, three teaspoons of cinnamon, whipped cream and only a trace of cinnamon - or better - a couple of blurps of Bailey's. Blend till smooth, share and enjoy. Don't waste this on kids, this is for adults!

RECIPES 10: ORANGE SCONES-HOW TO MAKE SCONES

All wants to learn how to make scones ...

You can either make them from scratch, or use a blend.

There's nothing like a moist delicious morning scone. You should also go along with any of many combinations to make them. This will encourage you to have light and flaky scones without attempting to find the right combination of ingredients all by yourself.

What are scones?

They are wonderful pastries, eaten more often at brunch, but good with tea or coffee at any time. They are particularly popular in England but can be found in many forms around the world.

They are a fast growing item in America as well. Some Bakeries, delis and bed & Breakfasts are beginning to serve them to the delight of their customers and guest.

Traditional scones are easy to make and many recipes build off of the basic method for baking that you are about to learn. Most of the recipes you will find flavors like orange, orange cranberry, blueberry, apricot and cream that find their beginnings in this basic scone mix.

Basic Ingredients

You can still change to scone baking mixes for a little support, as mentioned earlier, but this is not really important. With a simple recipe you can make English scones which are fast and convenient. Simple scones find their start in dry ingredients such as baking powder.

Typical dry ingredients include baking powder, baking soda, sugar, salt and flour but these simple ingredients can also differ. This also contains milk or buttermilk, bacon, and butter. You'll want to preheat your oven before you start the job, so that it's ready when your dough is.

The Mixing Process

These simple scones are made by mixing the dry ingredients together first and then cutting the butter into this dry mixture. When the butter is cut in cold instead of merely being mixed in, then it maintains a form of small lumps which help to make them light and flaky when they are done baking.

The milk or buttermilk and eggs are separately mixed and then added to the butter and dry ingredients. This mixing is continued until the resulting dough is somewhat lumpy.

It's important to remember that you don't want to add so much of the dough or that it may be hard for you. It's a technique mastered with practice. The dough is cut into triangles and then placed onto a baking sheet to complete the process of making the scone.

Anyone who wants to know how to make them will make those simple delicacies. The particulars are left out as they are rendered a bit differently everywhere you go. When you try to recreate the scone you've enjoyed in one place so you deserve to get your hands on the local recipe.

Using Scone Mixes

Mixes are my method of choice! If you eat scones on a regular basis you will realize that having a quick and easy preparation method is very important.

This approach usually tells you to cut it in cold butter and add the mixing kit to your mixing pot. Blend together those two things.

Load 1 cup of milk into a mixing cup and add an egg, then blend together with a fork. Pour the mixture into the bowl over the mixture and blend with a large spoon. Place a spoonful in a scone jar, or put it on an ungreased cookie sheet. Put them into the preheated oven for 12-14 minutes.

Orange Poppy Seed Scone Recipe

The orange poppy seed scone recipe has a zesty citrus taste. Great for an anytime of the day snack!

- o Ingredients
- o 2 1/4 cups all-purpose flour
- o 1/2 cup granulated sugar
- o 1/4 cup poppy seeds
- o 1 teaspoon cream of tartar
- o 3/4 teaspoon baking soda
- o 1/2 teaspoon salt
- o 1 stick (1/2 cup) unsalted butter, chilled
- o 1/4 cup orange juice
- o 1 large egg
- o 1/2 teaspoon grated orange peel

Egg Wash:

- o 1 egg
- o 1/2 teaspoon water

- ○ Hardware
- ○ Whisk
- ○ Large bowl
- ○ 2 x small bowls

Pastry blender (optional)

Pastry brush

Cookie sheet

Step 1: Preheat oven to 375 degrees F.

Step 2: Lightly grease a 10-inch diameter circle in center of cookie sheet; set aside.

Step 3: In a large bowl, whisk together flour, sugar, poppy seeds, cream of tartar, baking soda, and salt.

Step 4: With a pastry blender or knife cut in chilled butter until mixture resembles coarse crumbs.

Step 5: In a small bowl, stir together the orange juice, egg, and grated orange peel.

Step 6: Pour juice mixture into flour mixture and stir to combine.

Step 7: With lightly floured hands, pat dough into an 9-inch diameter circle in center of prepared cookie sheet.

Step 8: In a small bowl, stir together egg and 1/2 teaspoon water. Lightly brush egg mixture over the top of scones.

Step 9: With a serrated knife cut circle into 8 wedges.

Step 10: Bake 20-25 minutes or until set and lightly browned. Do not overbake. Re-cut wedges with knife. Let scones stand for 3 minutes before transferring to cooling surface.

Whole Grain Cranberry Orange Scones

These delicious scones are perfect for breakfast or afternoon tea. Not only are the whole grains included to provide nutritional value; they actually add a savory nutty background flavor that suits the honey and orange flavours.

A food processor is the perfect method for producing scone recettes. For you it does all the hard work, and with better results than hand-made ones.

Ingredients for 12 scones:

- o 10 ounces whole wheat flour (that's about 2 1/4 cups)
- o 4 teaspoons aluminum-free baking powder
- o 1/4 teaspoon baking soda
- o 1/4 teaspoon sea salt
- o 2 tablespoons extra virgin olive oil
- o 2 tablespoons cold butter (1/2 stick), or solid vegetable shortening
- o 1 tablespoon finely shredded orange zest
- o 2 tablespoons honey
- o 3/4 cup milk
- o 1 cup dried cranberries, roughly chopped

Directions:

Preheat oven to 400 F. In the food processor work bowl equipped with either a multipurpose blade or dough blade, mix the whole wheat flour, baking powder, baking soda, and salt. Pulse a couple of times until it mixes well. Stir in the olive oil and pump until all blended. Break or shorten the butter into small cubes, then add. Pulse a few more times before little peas are as large as chocolate.

Stir in the milk the honey and orange zest, then combine well. Switch the food processor on and slowly drizzle through the feed tube over the milk mixture. Stop when added to scarcely. In the cranberries use a spatula to fold gently.

Turn the dough onto a floured board or countertop and split into two pieces. Quickly work each into a circle, about 3/4 inch thick, dusting lightly with flour if it is too sticky to work with. Cut each circle into 6 even pie shaped wedges and transfer to a baking sheet lined with parchment paper. Bake for 12 - 16 minutes, or until golden brown.

Tips and Suggestions

Serve with fresh melted butter for a nice treat (it's simpler than you know with a food processor!) If you like extra sugar, sprinkle with the honey.

When making every pastry there are a variety of things to hold in mind. Your dough has to be cool to stop premature melting of the fat. At the very least, that means your butter must be well chilled. Chilling the flour also is recommended on warm days. Over-mixing makes a difficult scone. If the wet and dry components are combined, be sure to add as least as is completely required.

RECIPES 11:   DEVILED EGGS-A BRIEF HISTORY OF DELICIOUS DEVILED EGGS

Since no one can remember there were eggs around. The endless question always comes up, "What did the chicken or the egg come first?" In truth, all this really doesn't matter, because the fact is that the world loves them and has liked them for a very long time. Eggs can be fried in all manner of ways but deviled eggs must be the preference of the region. How did these very special eggs get produced and with whom?

First, we'll talk about the eggs' own existence to understand the origin of the deviled eggs themselves. They are certainly easy to get, used in many recipes and perfect for vegetarian people. Actually there are accounts of Jungle fowl being domesticated in India as from 3200 BC, China as from 1400 BC, the Romans came along shortly thereafter, and eventually domesticated fowl in North America with a Colombus voyage in 1493. The laying of eggs came along with the domestication and were all for our enjoyment. Back in the day the people did not eat only chicken eggs, there was all kinds of bird and mammal eggs like alligators.

The world can actually only suppose about when the use of eggs in baking started. The domestication of fowl had to start it, which was right about 6,000 BC (as discussed before). Historians do know that the making of breads and cake using eggs were made famous by Ancient Egyptian and Roman people. It was used as a thickening agent possibly by the use of trial and error. Nobles and priests in Egypt were having eggs in all their dishes.

Now it's on to the background of those tasty devilish eggs. Although eggs themselves have a very enigmatic history, for deviled eggs it must be believed that the same is true. They have no details. Though you may claim that it was something that was conceived in Ancient Rome. They became known to the Romans as Andalusia. In the 18th century, the word "deviled eggs" was coined. They will cook the eggs in Ancient Rome, and then serve them on top of spices. The eggs were used with everything from wine, pine kernels, celery, fish sauce, sugar, white vinegar, and pine nuts. That's a list of some very potent ingredients.

It also included stuffed eggs in medieval cookbooks. Within, there were raisins, goat cheese, marjoram basil, cloves and cinnamon. With all the ingredients in the same mix, you can imagine how those eggs tasted. Yeah! Just cool! Hard boiled eggs by the late 16th century had been all the rage. Then the hard-boiled egg became a staple in households by the 17th century.

It was the 18th century, when food started to "devil." It wasn't usually eggs that were devilled in the beginning. This is said that this is called "devilled" rice, since it is a fiery dish and thus similar to the extreme temperatures in which the devil (in hell) resides.

The recipes may all be slightly different, but my run ins with deviled eggs have all been pretty good so far. While it is a delicately simple appetizer, it packs a delicious punch, too. So put on those devilish medieval eggs and scatter the fat, or sugar, or flavour....whatever your heart desires. It is a game for everyone.

"Deliciously Fluffy Deviled Egg Platter" * Ingredients: 8 hard boiled eggs, 4 minced pickles, salt, pepper, 2 tsp of mustard Dijon, 1 tsp of chopped parsley, 1 cup of whipped cream, 2 tbs of buttermilk, 1/2 cup of chopped basil leaves, and 3 tbs of mayo.

1) Blend the whipped cream and buttermilk together. Cover with plastic wrap, and let stay for 8 hours or until dense at room temperature.

Possibly Page Split 2) Peel the eggs and cut in lengthwise direction. Then gently scrape the yolks with a knife. Put 4 yolks in a pot, and 4 yolks in a cup. Set the blanks back. Mash with a fork on any bowl of yolks.

2) Place the basil and mayo in a food processor. Blend for 2 minutes. Add the mixture to one bowl of yolks and mix. Then season with pepper and salt.

4) Add the crème mixture (crème fraiche), mustard, parsley, and pickles to the second bowl of yolks and mix. Season with salt and pepper.

5) Fill 4 of the egg whites with the first mixture and then fill the other 4 with the second mixture.

6) Enjoy with all the love of its mysterious history.

Deviled Eggs Recipe

Deviled eggs are perfect for a casual holiday meal or a pot luck party. They seem to be a favorite appetizer for tasty, relaxing, and party. Nothing is cooler than having a large batch and snacking on a handful before you set them out at the dinner party or pick them up for a picnic. Below is a short and basic recipes for deviled eggs, which can easily be made a few days ahead. So if you're up for a dumb, crowd-pleasing recipe then get your tools together and let's get started.

Hard-Cooking Eggs

The first step toward getting these simple deviled eggs is hard-cooking. A lot of people say hard-boil, but that is not the best word because, as you'll see, you're not really boiling them. They will be cooked over high heat until the water starts to boil and then is removed and left to stand until finished. Never leaving them to cook your eggs! If eggs are cooked for some amount of time, the yolks may become hard or can turn greenish-gray or unattractive.

Simply placed the eggs in a pan roomy enough to accommodate them without crowding, with at least one inch of cool water to cover with. First, heat up the water and eggs over high heat until they boil full. When a full boil is achieved, remove the saucepan from the flame, firmly cover it and let it stand for 15 minutes. Before that drain the hot water and run it for 5 minutes under cold water to avoid the cooking process. Placed them in the refrigerator at this stage to cool for a few hours. It should make peeling them faster.

Easy Deviled Eggs Recipe

- 12 hard boiled eggs
- 1/2 cup of mayonnaise
- 1 teaspoon prepared mustard
- 1/4 teaspoon salt
- 1/8 teaspoon cayenne
- 1 tablespoon curry powder

Now it is time for the deviled eggs to be made. After you peel them and cut them in half lengthwise, remove the yolks and place them in a bowl. This move is optional but to get them real good, you should run the yolks through a hand sifter. It makes for a deviled creamier potato.

Alternatively, just pound them with a fork. First, add all the other ingredients up to the yolks and combine well.

The final move is to take the mixture and place it in a container for food preservation. What you're going to do next is snip a hole into the corner of the bag and pip yolk mixture into white halves of the eggs. This is the fastest and cleanest way to get the deviled eggs ready for delivery.

There are a variety of variants to try, but I see this recipe for deviled eggs as the best tasting. It's easy to make, just take a couple of minutes to bring together, minus the cooking time for the eggs and let them cool down until they peel.

And if you want to get together when the group or family hit, then try this tasty and simple deviled egg recipe.

RECIPES 12:   GRANOLA BARS

Homemade granola bars are great treats every day – as part of a nutritious meal, afternoon snack, or lunch bag treat. Homemade recipes make granola bars so much savorer and safer, and less expensive from a box than the brand. Creating your own from scratch is truly fast. You can select from a wide range of recipes in cookbooks, food magazines, and directories on internet recipe.

Everyone loves granola bars but have you noticed they're so easy and inexpensive to make at home? When making homemade granola bars, you can change the taste and texture to suit your particular tastes and you can make them as tasty or decadent as you like. The recipe is very simple and needs only a few minutes of preparation hands followed by a fast hike through the oven. At the end you've got a big tray of delicious treats that will keep you warm for at least a week in a hot pool.

Both granola bars are a basic mixture of rolled oats, starch, sweetener, fat and add ins like; dried fruit, almonds, beans, spices, chocolate chips, pretzel bits, flaked coconut or puffed grains. By designing them yourself you get to pick just what you want to bring in and how much you want to bring in. You can select your own favorite combinations of flavors, or you can clone the combinations of flavors from your favorite popular brands. You can produce entirely new flavors and textures by playing with ingredients.

Using different ingredients like popcorn, pretzels or puffed grains can change the finished bar's appearance in fresh and unforeseen ways. You may also choose to apply ingredients slightly to adjust the final result, for example by not applying chocolate chips to the mix instead of waiting for the finished tray to come out of the oven and dumping the chips over the top of the granola. The leftover heat from the granola will melt the chocolate chips easily and you can then thinly scatter the chocolate over the top of the granola. The chocolate will re-harden when the granola cools, giving you a chocolate-coated granola bar, instead of a granola bar with chocolate chips inside. Even if the ingredients are the same, merely modifying where you add the chocolate makes the flavor special.

It makes organic granola bars great for Gluten Intolerance, Dairy Allergies, Protein Allergies and Soy Allergies. Whether you have a food limit or allergy, it's easy to skip the foods that bother you. If you have children, you can make a tasty and nutritious snack for their lunch bags or if you want an alternative to excessively sweet chocolate bars you can throw in tiny quantities of chocolate such as mini-M & Ms and make them into a granola / candy mix that suits both you and your children.

The quality of home-made granola bars vs. store-bought is that you can skip the frequently used artificial colors, fillers, additives and preservatives of professionally packaged products. You should be relaxed realizing that it is both safe and good for your family to enjoy your nice tasting, home-made snacks and that you get the best out of your food budget.

The Granola bars come in many different types and flavors. Some men are chewy; some are crunchy. Others have long product lists and some have only a handful. Some are calling for packaged granola while others are calling for that granola such as rolled oats, almonds, fruits and a number of sweeteners.

The key is to find a recipe that is right for you in a flavor and style. It is important to note that recipes are supposed to be a reference and when making homemade granola bars you can feel free to play. If a recipe includes raisins, and you'd like dried cherries, make the move. Baking is intended to be enjoyable and imaginative, if it makes sense for the substitutions, such as one kind of fruit or nut to another.

If you've ever wondered how to make granola bars, just how simple they are would impress you. Homemade granola bar recipes, like many bar-cookie recipes, are only safer and faster. Most contain dried fruits and nuts and rarely call for whole-wheat meals. Some are likely to bake and others are not.

Sometime ago a friend told me about the health benefits of dark chocolate lately and became a fan by applying it to a great granola recipe. I purchased the balls and the squares and the circles. The Coins are the most valuable of all. Semi-sweet morsels of chocolate have less fat and sugar than some other brands of chocolate and also fulfill my cravings; after all, dark chocolate is a modern health food. Look it up! No joke.

- o 1/3 c. safflower oil
- o 1 c. wild, raw honey
- o 1/2 tsp. salt
- o 1/2 tsp. vanilla extract
- o 5-6 c. old-fashioned rolled oats (not instant)
- o 1 c. wheat germ
- o 2 c. unsalted pumpkin seeds
- o 1/2 c. walnuts or cashews
- o 1/2 c. brown sugar (optional)
- o 1 c. semi-sweet chocolate morsels
- o 2 c. golden raisins or other dried fruits

Preheat oven to 300o F and line two, 12"x18 "rimmed parchment paper baking sheets, then spray with non-stick cooking oil.

Mix dried foods together: barley, wheat germ, pumpkin seeds, brown sugar and nuts.

Combine the honey (in this dish you can use almost any honey), the safflower oil and salt in a shallow saucepan over medium heat. Here's a trick: If you gently oil the mixing cup you're using with the sugar, it'll quickly come out.

Remove to dry, and blend well. The mixture of honey will be moist enough to pour in safely. Add vanilla and then whisk. Pour moist mixture of honey over the oat mixture and whisk until well powdered.

Place the mixture on the prepared baking sheets and roast, stirring for about 35 minutes at 15 minutes intervals until toasted and dark golden in color. Watch carefully to stop flames. Granola won't look crispy until it absolutely cools off.

When you find your simple recipe prototype, you'll be on your way to making a tasty home-made nutritious snack that you can enjoy day or night at any time.

RECIPES 13:   THAI SAUCE, PAD THAI RECIPE, AND THAI CURRY RECIPE

Two items depend on the secret to Thai food: Thai Herbs and Thai Sauce. Herbs are all about the fragrance but the sauce comes from the mouth watering flavor. Delicious Thai dishes come from great recettes of Thai sauce. If you have the correct mix you're on your way to great Thai Food cooking.

Look over to your neighbors' table next time you find yourself in a Thai restaurant. Often in those dishes, you will find small extra Thai sauces, unless your particular Thai restaurant serves non-Thais in particular. The more Thai sauces you see at tables the more authentic Thai food you'll get, I think what I'm saying is. It's generally a positive thing when such sauces taste nice on the tiny plates. You may presume the other sauces actually come from sauce recipes which are well produced. Best still, you know this restaurant is pretty authentic if you see condiments with Thai sauce and spices on the menu. Thai cuisine is about bringing together the vegetables, ingredients, and sauces. There is no better way than thai sauce to offer all the strong flavors. Thai sauce is split into two categories: sauce to eat and sauce to dunk in.

Thai Sauces:

Dipping Sauce • Prik Naam Pla (sliced chili and lime juice fish sauce)-a common sauce that goes with almost every rice dish. It was included in the condiment at several restaurants.

• Prik Naam Som (chili & vinegar sauce)-seasoning for flavoring noodles • Naam Prik Pao (roasted chili paste)-seasoning used in a number of dishes (soups, salads, stir frites). Some Thais use Nam Prik Pao to spread on toast as a replacement for jam.

• Aa-jaad (pickled cucumber salad)-fantastic fried fish cakes dipping sauce, satay and other fried appetizers

• Naam Jiem Saate (peanut sauce)-one of Thailand's most popular out-side sauces. It tastes so good people not only use it to dip Satay but use it as a salad dressing, substitute for pizza sauce, substitute for pad thai sauce and much more. The American ought to name it "What Milk" sauce, whatever meal you what dipping in that sauce.

• Naam Jiem Talay (Seafood Sauce)-you guessed it, right. Naam Jiem Talay is a dipping sauce to match your desires for seafood. Step over chocolate! Have your mouth open for a fiesta. This bad boy is full of flavor, and the strong mix of spicy, sour, salty, and sweet can blow off your socks until you take a bite.

• Naam Jiem Buoi (Plum sauce)-popular with children and those unable to stomach spicy food. Nam Jiem Buoi is perfect for any form of fried rice.

• Jig Choe (vinaigrette soy sauce)-use to make hot and sour soup and to dip pot sticker sauce and Dim Sum.

• Naam Jiem Gai (sauce for chicken dipping)-soft, spicy sauce. Great with BBQ chicken • Naam Jiem Seir Rong Hai (cry tiger sauce)-Crying tiger is one of the most popular American dishes. Seared medium rare beef eaten with dipping sauce, composed of fish sauce, ground roasted rice, chilli pepper, soy sauce, and lime juice. Cooking Sauce

• Pla nam (fish sauce)-to add spicy flavour. Stir fry in soups, and make sauces. In dishes such as Tom Yum (hot and sour soup), Tom Kah (coconut soup), and pad krapow (stir fry, holy basil) you can find fish sauce.

• Nam Som Sai Choo (vinegar)-for bitter flavouring. Using sweet and sour stir fry in soups.

• Thai Pad Sauce-Use for Thai pad preparation. Our later post will highlight Pad Thai recipe.

• Phu Khao Tong (soy sauce with a green lid)-soy sauce with flavour. One of the essential sauces that many Thai stir fry sauce recipes included

• See Dum (Sweet black soy sauce)-for making Pad See iew (Sweet sir fried chinese broccoli and meat noodle).

Khao Mun Khai ingredient (Broiled chicken meat over flavored rice) dipping sauce • See khao view (light soy sauce)-essential sauce in other dipping sauce.

• Tammarin juice-a major ingredient in thai pad sauce. Included in some dipping sauce and Thai Khang Som soup (Sour tammarin based broth) • Oyster sauce-ingredient in many Thai stir fry sauce recettes like sweet and sour fry swirl.

• Curry paste-There are common herbs and spices in both curry pastes but different proportions.

Thai Curry recipe will be given in our later article.

- o Green curry paste
- o Yellow curry paste
- o Red curry paste
- o Mussamun curry paste
- o Chu chee curry paste
- o Panang curry paste
- o Khua Kling curry paste (Southern Thai food)
- o Khang Pa curry paste (Not popular in foreign country)
- o Khang Som curry paste (Not popular in foreign country)

As it's clearly written above, the majority of Thai food relies on Thai sauce. When you combine the sauces and balance them, they are entirely different dishes.

Even the same recipes make a major difference in flavor, with varying proportions. That's why sauce recettes are the secret to distinguishing decent Thai food from excellent Thai delicacy.

Like I said, "When you have the correct mix, you're on the road to great Thai food cooking."

Who Loves Cooking in Thai?

We are! And we hope that you do that too-or, at least we hope that you will soon! Anyway, Local Thai Food is run by only a few of us locals here in Southern California and we would love to serve you!

Which Food for Thais?

That is a big issue. Now that's a perfect comment here: we prefer Thai cuisine. Okay, we love Thai food really. And we love Thai food so much we think you will also enjoy it. And so, it's our mission to offer a simple and convenient way to find the food they love to anyone who loves Thai food-or anyone who loves food in general.

What Is Thai Local Food?

The answer is quite simple: spicy and delicious Thai food, you can smell it so close! Okay, maybe not near enough but near enough to stuff yourself with fantastic food

RECIPES 14:   HEALTHY DESSERTS

I must confess I was extremely doubtful when I first came across the notion that you would turn the basic ingredients of banana and flax into cookies. How will a cookie be baken without flour, baking powder or cookie dough? Because I try in my diet to eliminate these additives and stay clear of gluten and fried foods, this suggestion sounds too promising to be true. Of course I was really interested.

To claim that my first few attempts at producing a cookie using bananas from scratch was a failed experiment is an understatement. Many websites tell you to bake them for 10-11 minutes. This never worked. I also kept having problems with an extremely runny batter. After some time it seemed like a tasty cookie without the usual ingredients just wasn't going to happen.

The eureka moment recently occurred in my kitchen, however. And with a few secrets and adjustments to the recipes already out there, it can happen in yours too.

What you need for the perfect batter:

- o   3 ripe bananas
- o   5-6 teaspoons of flaxseed meal (I use Bob's Red Mill)
- o   4-5 tablespoons of honey

- 2-3 tablespoons of egg white (THIS is the secret ingredient)

Mash the bananas into a smooth, even consistency with a fork and/or whisk in. When this is performed manually, it is possible to leave tiny bits in the batter for tastier cookies. Add the remaining ingredients, then add a bit of white egg. That will fix a runny batter's problem altogether.

The next trick is to use greased parchment paper with extra virgin olive oil. Take a paper towel and rub the oil on it, then uniformly scatter on parchment paper. With this paper line a 13 x 9 aluminum baking pan.

Eventually, keep a close watch on baking temperature and cooking time. I haven't had any luck with recipes asking for 12 minutes of baking at 350 The cookies were almost never finished. After some trials I find that 375 and 35 minutes was the right figures. Simply spoon the batter into thin, uniformly spaced mounds, and bake for about 35 minutes uncovered on the center oven rack.

The cookies can get incredibly crisp at 40 minutes and beyond, so track them carefully to match your taste. When they're finished baking, require them to cool for 20 minutes in the pan and on top of the stove.

Follow those easy secrets and you will have cookies that are incredibly tasty (and amazingly healthy). The above proportions will make about 15-20 cookies. For smaller batches use 1.5 teaspoons of flaxseed meal for every one banana. And always remember to use some egg white! This is an easy recipe to master, and will leave you with delicious, grain free, all natural desserts that are full of potassium and omega-3 and entirely free of processed food.

What's more, I have yet to meet a child that doesn't love these. Happy baking!

Banana flaxseed cookies are also quite versatile for some additional flavorings and ingredients.

Make Healthier Chocolate Chip Cookies

Is it possible to indulge in healthy chocolate chip cookies which taste good from time to time? Sure, and to show it, I've picked a dozen recipes for healthy chocolate chip cookies.

Most "balanced cookies" don't taste so well so, I don't think the calories are worth it.

After a lifetime of weight challenges, I discovered that every now and then I'd rather have a little, delicious cookie than a bunch of tasteless replacements, even though they're supposed to be good. I am a survivor of the "Snackwells" era, where I was somehow persuaded without remorse that I should eat tons of such tasteless wonders. I managed to gain weight even though I got zero gratification!

I'm mature now, and a little bit smarter. I know what works for me-good diet, organic food. So I'm searching for remedies when it comes to indulgences that will please my taste buds so my need for balanced goodness.

It's important to note that a cookie with chocolate chips is an indulgence to eat sparingly. It can never be a completely nutritious product, and can only be made too good before it starts losing its lusciousness.

How to Make Chocolate Chip Cookies Healthier?

There are a lot of things you can do to make cookies healthier and improve their quality. Here are a few of my favorites: use less fat or a healthy fat Replacement part of the fat with applesauce or yogurt Replace all or some of the flour with whole wheat or other whole grain flour Add some beans, almonds, seeds and/or dried fruit Add some ground flaxseed Use dark chocolate chips Replace all or part of the sugar with a natural sweetener such as honey, maple syrup, brown rice syrrringe

Attach a wholesome fruit or vegetable such as sliced zucchini, mashed bananas, or pumpkin puree.

Almond Butter Chocolate Chip Cookies Recipe Makes about 24 cookies These cookies have a lot to do with them-low in calories, free from dairy, free from gluten, simple and tasty. We easily mix together with only 6 ingredients and you can eat luscious, moist chocolate chip cookies from the oven in 30 minutes or less. They are asking for Sucanat-dehydrated cane juice-but then, you can use plain brown sugar.

- o 1 cup almond butter
- o 3/4 cup Sucanat
- o 1 large egg
- o 1/2 teaspoon baking soda
- o 1/4 teaspoon sea salt
- o 3 ounces dark chocolate (at least 70%), broken into small pieces

Preheat oven to 350F. Cover parchment baking sheets or silicone liners.

In a medium dish, whisk in the almond butter, sucanat, sugar, baking soda and salt until mixed. Stir in the candy pieces before combining them in the mixture.

Fall rounded spoons of cookie dough on lined baking sheets leaving about 2 inches between cookies. Bake for 10 to 12 minutes, or until lightly browned. Remove from the oven and cool down on baking sheets for 5 minutes, then pass cookies to wire racks for another 15 minutes to cool.

RECIPES 15:   PICKLES-PICKLED VEGETABLES FOR SALADS

My favorite vegetables are English cucumbers, carrots and cauliflower for these fresh and savory vegetable pickles. They are sliced in chunks, with a lovely soft sour taste, very finely pickled. Perfect as finger food for casual fun, they last in the refrigerator for up to a week.

I have always made these and have used different quantities of vegetables so I don't have a set ingredient formula. I offer the basic guidance and you will be guided by individual tastes. I like sweet pickles, maybe some don't. I like the flavor of pickling seasoning, maybe you don't.

• The carrots are better washed and sliced into around 21/2 cm thick chunks.

• The coliflower will split into tiny flowers.

• All vegetables would have as much freshness as possible.

• Drop the cooked carrots and coliflower into easily boiling water before the water returns to the boil, drain and then placed in another cold water container to avoid the boiling process. This is called par-boiling and they are crisply half cooked and ready to be pickling afterwards.

• English cucumbers are not peeled, cut into chunks or thinly sliced, seasoned with salt to eliminate excess moisture and drained after around 10 minutes until they have become very limp.

• Pickling paste for cucumber slices: blend hot water, sugar and vinegar to taste and pour over the slices of the cucumber. It can just be slightly sweet-sour, because you are cooking a salad and not a real pickle. It will last in the fridge coated in the pickling brine for around a week.

• Pickling mixture for carrots and coliflower: Boil water, sugar and vinegar together in the same proportion as in step 3 and then apply pickling spice, shut off the stove and let the mixture steep until tender. Then spill over the carrots and cauliflower, and refrigerate in their brine for up to a week.

Note: These finely pickled vegetables maintain their flavor and are very enticing They are often tasty when added to snack platters and frozen meats at weddings or on a small scale at cocktail parties or bring-a-plate events like PTA meetings and barbecues.

Consider it your strength and you'll never scratch your head on whether to take to a social event again, because everyone looks forward to your tasty vegetables!

The slices of pickled cucumber are perfect on cold meat sandwiches, can be added to a green salad, or eaten alone as salad.

Bread and Butter Pickles Are you having a barbecue, dreaming about the right food items to bring? When you want a nutritious snack that is easy to make and tastes fantastic, try to prepare pickles with the bread and butter.

The sweet-sour food is absolutely wonderful. The perfect mix of ingredients makes it absolutely appetizing and scrumptious. You can eat the pickles straight from the bottle, or use them as sandwich or hamburger toppings. Pasta salads and cold beef with these pickles mixed in, will also taste great.

Many shops sell pickles from bread and butter; in the store you can find them readily available in airtight cans. You can do these pickles with too much ease though. Below are simple measures to help you make the finest sweet and sour pickles.

1. Prepare the needed ingredients.

Sweet and sour pickles contain cucumbers, tomatoes, vinegar, pickling oil, turmeric, mustard seeds, celery seeds and a few ice cubes.

2. Thinly slice the cucumbers and clean the pan to crisp.

Combine the onions and the sliced cucumbers into a metal pot. Load generous quantities of pickling salt onto the vegetables to enhance flavor. Then, put ice cubes on top to crisp the cucumbers. Cover the bottle, then set aside for several hours. This brining and crisping process can take overnight for the pickles to produce a better product.

3. Mix with the remaining components.

Taking off excess liquid after brining and crisping the cucumbers. Then clean the vegetables and wash. Layer the cucumbers, onion, and other ingredients in a large saucepan. Cook until nearly boiling. Before you hit the mixture boils make sure you steppe the cucumbers. Switch off heat and allow to cool down the ingredients for a while.

4. Place the ingredients in a pot.

When the vinegar and sugar have melted, add it into the frying pan. Throw in the onion and the cucumbers. Give up a little gap at the end. Then, place the open jars in a hot water tub. The cycle of hot canning destroys every organism in the container. Then, cover the jars and for several days you can put them in the fridge.

Like the other styles of pickles, bread and butter pickles take a limited period of time just to get in the flavor. Hence, after the canning cycle, you can eat it many hours. Use it for popular foods such as hamburgers, tacos, salads or frozen beef. You're likely to enjoy the recipe's sweet and sour flavor, which should appeal to sensitive taste buds.

You may also eat the pickles simple, which allows a nice snack that's low in calories. Weight-watchers and health-conscious individuals will love munching on the sugar and vinegar mixture on the crispy cucumbers. Seek to make pickles for bread and butter by following the simple steps set out in this e-book. You'll definitely have an simple time to make a fun snack food item that the whole family would enjoy.

I don't know about you, Daikon, Carrot & Cucumber Salad, but Japan is like hard work, commitment and technology for me, but I just found that their food is just as sweet. Japanese cuisine is rich in protein, since the main source of food is from the sea. Attempt the recipe below and I know you'd enjoy it.

Ingredients:

- o 450g (1 lb) daikon, peeled and sliced into thin lengths (about 3 cups), soaked in cold water for 10 mins and drained
- o Small Japanese cucumbers or pickling cucumbers (gherkins cut into long, thin strips. Stop before reach the seeds (about 2/3 cups)

- 1 small carrot
- 1 small onion
- Sheets of nori lightly toasted, halved and drained
- 3 tea spoons of black sesame seeds

Ingredients for Dressing:

- o 2 tablespoons soy sauce
- o 2 table spoons mirin
- o 1 teaspoon white sugar
- o 2 table spoons rice wine vinegar
- o 1 teaspoon dashi powder dissolved in 1 table spoon water

Method of preparation:

- o Blend all the ingredients in a big bowl and put aside to make the sauce.
- o To assemble salad, toss the daikons onion slices in a medium bowl, pile the tossed vegetables high on a medium serving plate, pour over the prepared dressing immediately before serving and top with roasted nori and sesame seeds

Remarks:

Nori

A type of seaweed pressed into thin sheets and baked (yaki nori) or seasoned with soy sauce (ajitsuke nori). It is sold in 23 x 17 cm (9 x 7 in) sheets and usually packed in bundles of 10. Ajisuke nori is served as appetizers while yaki nori is served with rice.

Dashi powder

Its the equivalent of the western soup stock powder. It is normally used to make dashi fish stock and as a basic seasoning in many Japanese recipes.

Delicious Egg Recipes

Eggs are delicious, incredibly versatile, and very healthy when eaten in moderation. Today the EZ Cracker Egg Separator makes egg cooking easier than ever before. It uses an innovative mechanism that helps you to break eggs in your food without making a mess or having shell bits. Often, the EZ Cracker comes with an extension so you can either separate the yolk from the white or remove the shells from a hard boiled egg.

Here are few delicious and savory egg recipes you should try today.

Huevos Rancheros

Huevos rancheros are a delicious Mexican-style breakfast that can easily lend itself to many different variations. This recipe is just a guideline. Feel free to eliminate toppings or add a few new ones of your own.

- 2 eggs
- 1 soft tortilla shell
- 1/2 avocado, sliced
- Refried beans
- Shredded Mexican cheese
- Salsa

- o Sour cream
- o Oil or cooking spray

Start by coating the bottom of a frying pan with a little bit of oil or a shot of cooking spray. Heat it up on high for a few seconds, and then crack two eggs directly into the pan. While they are starting to fry, put the tortilla on a plate and spread the refried beans onto it. Sprinkle some shredded Mexican cheese on top and throw it in the microwave until the cheese melts.

At this point you are going to want to flip the eggs. You can get out a spatula and do this but what is the fun in that? If you used the right amount of oil and the bottom of the egg is cooked enough you should be able to shake the pan and have the half-fried egg move around a little bit without separating. Give it a few shakes to loosen it up and then try to flip them into the air and onto the other side.

While the other side of the egg is cooking you can grab the tortilla out of the microwave and start adding the slices of avocado. Slide the fried eggs onto the center of the plate and then add the salsa and sour cream on top. Enjoy!

Indian Deviled Eggs

Deviled eggs are a classic and delicious appetizer. This recipe mixes it up by adding a dash of Indian flavor! It is also a little healthier than traditional deviled eggs because the mayonnaise has been eliminated.

- 6 hard-boiled eggs
- 1/2 large red onion, minced
- 1 tsp ground black pepper
- 1 tsp curry powder
- 3 tbsp fresh cilantro (also known as coriander), finely chopped
- Little bit of oil for frying
- Salt to taste
- Chutney for topping (optional)

After you have hard boiled the eggs, cut them in half lengthwise and carefully remove the yolk. Set aside the whites. Heat the oil in a pan and saute the onions until they turn clear. Stir in the pepper, curry, and cilantro. Once it is mixed well, add the egg yolks and mash it all up until it is smooth.

Notice we have yet to add the salt. A little bit of salt is essential for humans but we often tend to overdo it. Taste the mixture at this point and if it is good you can forgo the salt altogether. If not, stir in a little bit at a time until it suits your taste. Now you just carefully spoon the mixture back into the white. Top with your preferred chutney (mango chutney is delicious!) and serve. Viola!

Baked Vegetable Omelet

Omelets are an old egg standby. They are delicious and they are open to all kinds of variations. Here we mix things up a bit and bake the omelet instead of frying it. Baking almost always results in a fluffier and airy omelet.

This recipe calls for a variety of vegetables, but feel free to get creative with it by adding your own favorite ingredients. Makes enough to feed four people.

- o   1 cup shredded Monterey Jack Cheese
- o   2 cups shredded cheddar cheese
- o   2 cups broccoli, chopped
- o   3 tomatoes, chopped
- o   1 red onion, chopped
- o   1 1/3 cup milk
- o   1/3 cup flour
- o   1/2 tsp salt
- o   4 eggs

Start by heating the oven up to 350 degrees. Then layer the Jack cheese, vegetables, and cheddar in a square baking dish. 8"x8x2 is ideal.

Now beat the eggs with the milk, flour and salt until it is smooth and pour it over everything else. Then just bake for about 45 minutes, starting to check at about 30 to see how the egg mixture is setting. Let it cool for ten minutes and then serve it up!

These are just a few of the many egg recipes made easier with the EZ Cracker Egg Separator. And remember that these recipes are just the guidelines. There are no set rules to cooking.

Avocado

Known as one of the most versatile fruit, avocado can either be cooked or eaten raw. In some countries like the Philippines, Indonesia, Vietnam and Brazil, avocado is enjoyed as a dessert drink mixed with milk, sugar and water. Mexico and Central America enjoys this fruit as a part of the main dish served with rice, salads, chicken and meat. Jamaicans enjoy this alongside bread or bulla.

Vegetarian chefs do prefer to substitute meat with avocado, as the former has a high fat quality. This good-tasting fruit is also perfect for making rolls and maki sushi in California. Apart from its rich texture and flavor, avocado is high in potassium, vitamins B and vitamin E. It also provides a strong source of protein and carbohydrates. On the other hand, avocado oils are rich in lecithin, antioxidants and vitamins A and E which help maintain healthy and youthful skin. The antioxidants present in this fruit help to fend off cancer cells while at the same time helping to keep the skin clear of wrinkles.

Are you low on budget? Here is a simple way for you to enjoy home-made avocado beauty products. To make an avocado facial, you will need 1/2 cup non-instant oatmeal, 1 cup mashed avocado and 1 to 2 tablespoons honey. Just mix all the ingredients in a blender and blend it until it becomes smooth. Apply it to your face. Let it dry for 15 minutes, rinse and pat dry with a towel. This very easy and affordable spa-like home treatment will give your skin rejuvenation and reduce eye puffiness.

To have a thoroughly-cleansed skin, make an avocado deep cleanser. What you will need are 1 egg, 1/2 cup milk and 1/2 avocado which is already ripe and has been peeled. In a bowl, beat the egg yolk until it becomes light and frothy. Then, add milk and the avocado. Apply it to your skin using cotton just like you would do with other cleansers and enjoy the deep cleansing effect. This mixture is effective against pollutants and also good to use after cleansing your face with soap and water. Refrigerate any leftovers to preserve it.

CPSIA information can be obtained
at www.ICGtesting.com
Printed in the USA
BVHW011118080621
609002BV00002B/69